WORKBOOK TO ACCOMPANY

VANDER / SHERMAN / LUCIANO

HUMAN PHYSIOLOGY

MATTHEW J. KLUGER

LOUIS G. D'ALECY

Professors of Physiology
University of Michigan

WORKBOOK TO ACCOMPANY

VANDER / SHERMAN / LUCIANO

HUMAN PHYSIOLOGY

Second Edition

McGRAW-HILL BOOK COMPANY

New York St. Louis San Francisco Auckland Düsseldorf Johannesburg Kuala Lumpur London Mexico Montreal New Delhi Panama Paris São Paulo Singapore Sydney Tokyo Toronto

This book was set in Helvetica Light by Progressive Typographers.
The editors were William J. Willey, Thomas A. P. Adams, and Douglas J. Marshall; the designer was Scott Chelius; the production supervisor was Sam Ratkewitch.
The Murray Printing Company was printer and binder.

WORKBOOK TO ACCOMPANY
VANDER / SHERMAN / LUCIANO
HUMAN PHYSIOLOGY

ISBN 0-07-066956-2

234567890 DODO 783210987

Contents

Acknowledgments

The authors would like to thank the staffs of the Department of Educational Resources of the School of Dentistry and the Department of Physiology of the School of Medicine, University of Michigan for their assistance in the production of this manual, particularly: Elizabeth Hitch, Ruth Ashley, and Nancy Daley for materials production; James Schulz for artwork; Daniel Burns, Pat LePeak, Brent Martin, Nadia Hidayet, and Nancy Tomaro for materials coordination; and Theresa Flournoy, Michael Kahl, Lynnette Maloney, and Mary Nishimuta for final typing.

Matthew J. Kluger
Louis G. D'Alecy

How to Use This Workbook

Organization

You will note as you flip through this workbook that there are 18 chapters of study in human physiology corresponding to the 18 chapters in the text. Each of these chapters is divided into several modules. Each module should take approximately $\frac{1}{2}$ to $1\frac{1}{2}$ hours to complete. Within each module there are several sections: Objectives, Reading Assignment, Supplemental Materials, Exercises, and Self-Test. Each of these sections is described in full below.

The figures appearing in this workbook are numbered W-1 through W-85. All references to double-numbered figures (8-20, etc.) are figures that appear in Vander, Sherman, and Luciano: *Human Physiology,* second edition.

Objectives

The objectives section of each module contains a listing of the objectives you will be expected to achieve at the end of the module. Read each objective carefully *before* you begin the reading assignment. Concentrate on the portions of the reading that will help you most in completing the objectives. Because educational objectives reflect the aims of a particular course and the value systems of a specific teacher, no one set of objectives meets all requirements. Select from the lists those objectives which meet your needs, modifying them whenever appropriate.

It must be emphasized that the objectives are almost entirely of the cognitive type; few ask the student to manipulate the material extensively or use the information to predict answers to a new problem. This is not because we believe such objectives are unimportant, but rather because explicit answers to such questions are not to be found in the book. We would urge your instructors to add to these objectives additional ones which do tell the student the kinds of manipulations, deductions, predictions, etc., the student should be able to perform.

Reading Assignment

All reading assignments are from the text *Human Physiology,* second edition, by Vander, Sherman, and Luciano.

Supplementary Materials

Occasionally a module will contain material that cannot be mastered by reading the text. In this case, supplementary materials (in the form of diagrams, additional reading material, etc.) are provided with the module. Your instructor will inform you which supplementary materials you are responsible for learning.

Exercises

When the objectives indicate that a review of materials would be beneficial, exercises have been provided. These exercises serve a workbooklike function in that they may be completed with the help of the text and used for review before each test. Each exercise is followed by a number in parentheses which indicates the page in the text where help in solving the exercise may be found.

Self-Test

Each module ends in a self-test. When you feel you can achieve each of the objectives listed for the module, take the self-test. Complete the test at your leisure in a "testing" environment (no books, notes, or distractions). When you have answered as many of the questions as you can, check your answers using the key provided in the back of the book. Refer to the pages in your text (shown on the key in parentheses) for answers that you missed or were unsure about. Remember that the self-test only provides a sample of questions.

Basic Cell Functions

It is assumed that much of the material on basic cellular functions as presented in Chapters 1 through 4 in your text has been or will be learned in other courses (for example, biochemistry). The student should be familiar with the content indicated by the objectives in these units. Self-tests without exercises have been provided for these chapters. If you are unsure of your ability to accomplish the objectives listed, take the diagnostic self-test to determine where study is needed.

Module I:
Atoms and Molecules

Module II:
The Structure and Properties of Organic Molecules

CHEMICAL COMPOSITION OF THE BODY

CHAPTER 1

Module I: Atoms and Molecules

Objectives

Upon completion of this module, the student will be able to:

1. Describe the location of protons, electrons, and neutrons within an atom and the electrical charges associated with each particle.
2. Describe and differentiate among atom, molecule, polar molecule, and ion.
3. Differentiate between the distribution of electrical charges within an atom and the process of ionization which results in formation of ions and polar molecules.
4. Describe the process of chemical bond formation in relation to the formation of neutral, polarized, or ionized molecules.
5. Differentiate between the English and metric systems of measurement by comparing inch to centimeter, pound to kilogram, and quart to liter.
6. Define *atomic weight, molecular weight, concentration,* and *mole.*
7. List the four most common atoms in the body.
8. List the three states of matter and give examples of each in the body.
9. Describe the process of ionization that results in the formation of an acid and an acidic solution.
10. Define *solute* and *solvent;* give examples of each in the body.
11. Describe the properties of water as a solvent and describe why water is an ideal medium for chemical reactions.

Reading Assignment

Chap. 1, pp. 6–15.

Self-Test

Part I

Directions: Complete the following items in the space provided.

1. The ____liquid state____ is intermediate in terms of freedom of molecular movement between solid and gas states.
2. ____Water (H_2O)____ is the major molecule responsible for the liquid state in the body.
3. The dissolved molecule in a solution is known as the ____solute____.
4. Acids are molecules which give rise to ____hydrogen____ ions.

5. The acidity of a solution is determined by the concentration of
hydrogen ions.

Part II

Directions: Circle the correct answer(s).

1. Each of the following is commonly soluble in a water solvent *except* for

   a sodium ion. *b* alcohols.
   (*c*) fats. *d* salts.

2. Sodium chloride is completely dissolved in water.

   a The sodium chloride is the solvent.
   (*b*) In solution, sodium chloride exists as sodium and chloride ions.
   c The water in this example is the solute.

Part III

Directions: Circle T for true and F for false.

(T) F 1. A paper match is approximately 1 mm thick and 3 mm wide.
(T) F 2. An average person is approximately 170 to 180 cm tall.
T (F) 3. A proton and an electron are the same weight but are opposite in charge. → proton has 2000 times the mass of an electron
T (F) 4. In the normal body, water exists in all three states (liquid, gas, and solid).
(T) F 5. Water is one of the end products of many chemical reactions in the body.
T (F) 6. Water is a good solvent for all the compounds in the body.
T (F) 7. All hydrogen-containing compounds are considered acids. → only those that ionize to form Hydrogen ions
T (F) 8. The formation of a chemical bond can only give rise to a neutral compound. → neutral polarized or ionized
(T) F 9. Both organic and inorganic acids are found in the body.
(T) F 10. The cells of the body are generally measured in micrometers.

Module II: The Structure and Properties of Organic Molecules

Objectives

Upon completion of this module the student will be able to:

1. Define and differentiate among inorganic, organic, and biochemistry.
2. Describe the general properties of a carbon atom and explain why an entire field of chemistry is devoted to its study.
3. Describe the general characteristic structure of proteins, lipids, and carbohydrates.
4. Identify the hydroxyl, carboxyl, amino, and phosphate chemical groups.
5. Describe the primary structure of a protein molecule using the terms polymer, amino acid, amino group, carboxyl group, and peptide bond.
6. List three functional roles played by proteins.
7. Describe the three-dimensional shape of various proteins.
8. Describe the three subclasses of lipids in terms of structure and give the physical property they have in common.
9. Define *monosaccharide, disaccharide,* and *polysaccharide* and give examples of these types of carbohydrates.
10. Differentiate between metabolism and metabolic intermediate.

Reading Assignment

Chap. 1, pp. 15–30.

Self-Test

Part I

Directions: Complete the following items in the space provided.

1. When a molecule of fatty acid contains *no* double bonds, it is said to be saturated.
2. The term used to refer to the class of molecules formed when all three hydroxyls in glycerol are substituted with fatty acids is neutral fat.

3. Inorganic chemistry is the chemistry of non-carbon molecules
4. A branch of organic chemistry relating specifically to living substances is biochemistry.
5. The liver can link many glucose units together to form glycogen which is classed as a(n) polysaccharides.
6. Sugars composed of two other sugars joined together are called disaccharides.
7. The term used to define the many chemical reactions normally occurring within the cell is metabolism.
8. As metabolism proceeds, many substances are formed which may or may not be related to the functioning of the cell. These substances are known as metabolic intermediates
9. The breakdown of carbohydrates to CO_2 and H_2O serves what function? provides major source of energy.

Part II

Directions: Circle the correct answer(s).

1. A peptide bond occurs between which two functional groups?

   a carboxyl and hydroxyl *b* amino and hydroxyl
   c two amino groups *d* amino and carboxyl

2. The primary structure of proteins refers to the

   a interaction of more than one peptide chain. c
   b alpha helix configuration.
   c sequence of amino acids.
   d random coiling prior to alpha helix formation.

3. Which of the following can be considered an organic compound?

   a sodium chloride *b* carbohydrates
   c calcium phosphate *d* hydrochloric acid

4. Which of the following describes the role(s) of protein in the body? Proteins

   a provide most of the chemical energy for the cells. b + c
   b are the primary component of connective tissue.
   c catalyze most chemical reactions in the body.
   d are necessary for energy storage.

5. Which of the following is the best reason why an entire field of chemistry is devoted to the study of carbon compounds? Carbon is

   a the most abundant atom in nature.
   b the only atom used by human cells.
   c able to form four separate bonds with other atoms.
   d unable to form bonds with other carbon atoms.

6. The body's most important monosaccharide is

   a galactose. *b* lactose.
   c glucose. *d* sucrose.

7. A common plant polysaccharide which the human body is unable to break down is

   a starch. *b* cellulose. *c* glycogen.

8. Which of the following comprise the basic components of a neutral fat molecule?

   a amino acids *b* fatty acids
   c glucose *d* ethanol
   e glycerol

9. Some hormones and cholesterol are common examples of

   a phospholipids. *b* proteins.
   c steroids. *d* fatty acids.

10. Because they contain both a polar and a nonpolar end, effective for water lipid interfaces, one of the following groups is a major component of cell membranes. Which one?

    a phospholipids *b* proteins
    c steroids *d* fatty acids
    e carbohydrates

Part III

Directions: The illustrations labeled A through E in Fig. W-1 are examples of the complete or partial structures of different classes of compounds. Match them with their correct names in the column below.

1. ________neutral fat
2. ________protein
3. ________steroid
4. ________phospholipid
5. ________carbohydrate

Match the terms in the left column with the correct chemical group shown on the right.

1. ________amino	A. OH
2. ________phosphate	B. NH_2
3. ________hydroxyl	C. COOH
4. ________carboxyl	D. PO_4

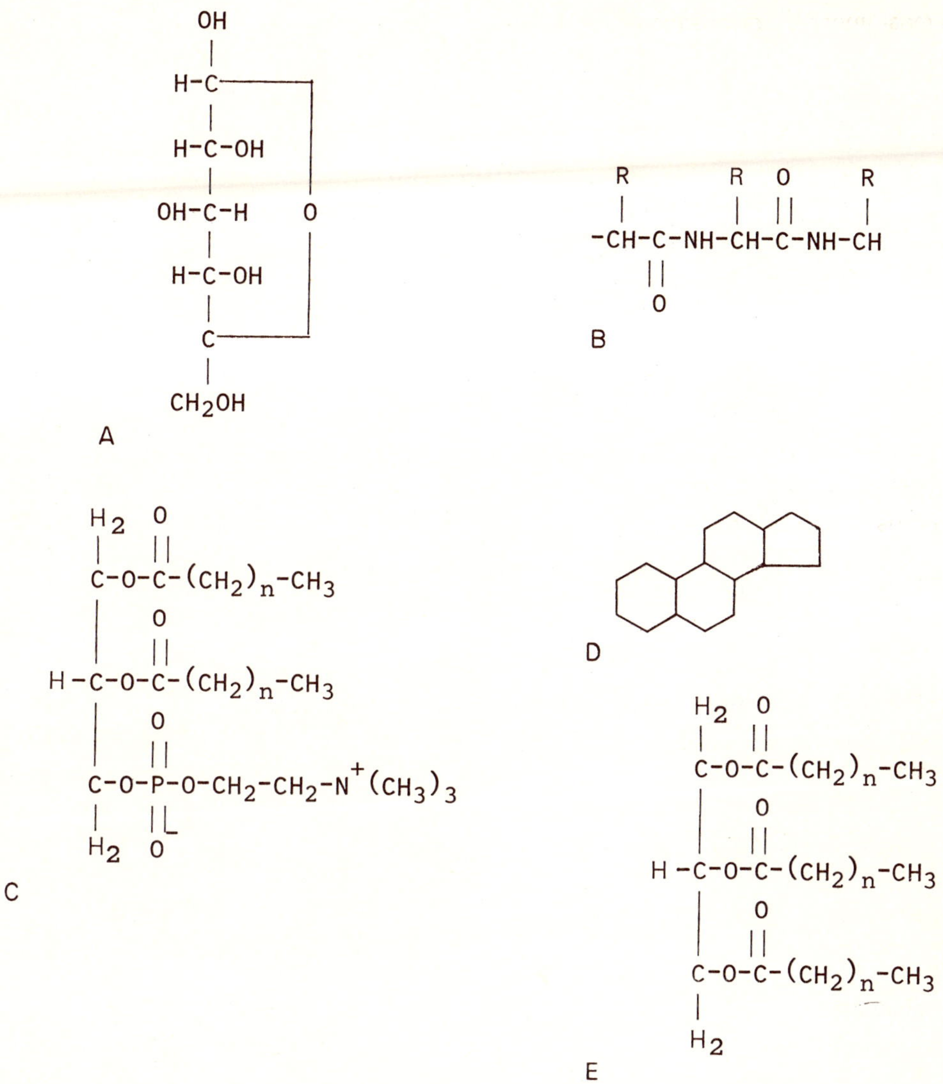

Fig. W-1

Module I:
The Cell, Bulk Flow, and Diffusion

Module II:
Mediated Transport and Osmosis

Module III:
Membrane Structure and Junction

CHAPTER 2 MOVEMENT OF MOLECULES ACROSS CELL MEMBRANES

Module I: The Cell, Bulk Flow, and Diffusion

Objectives

Upon completion of this module the student will be able to:

1. Describe the general structure of the cell in terms of membrane-bound chemical compartments using the terms protoplasm, organelles, Golgi apparatus, nuclear membrane, lipid droplets, ribosomes, secretion granules, nucleolus, mitochondria, and endoplasmic reticulum.
2. Define *semipermeable membrane* in terms of its role in governing the exchange of chemical compounds between cell and compartment.
3. Describe bulk flow and give examples of its occurrence in the three states of matter.
4. Define the driving force for bulk flow.
5. Write the equation for bulk flow and define each term of the equation.
6. Define diffusion in terms of the random movement of particles, net flux, and the dependence of diffusion on a concentration gradient.
7. Describe the effect of temperature on molecular motion.
8. Define *diffusion equilibrium* and *net diffusion.*
9. Write the equation for diffusion and define each term of the equation.
10. Write the equation for the net flux across a cell membrane and define each term in the equation.
11. Define *membrane permeability* and describe the relation of lipid solubility and molecular size to the permeability constant.
12. Differentiate between net flux and unidirectional flux, including a discussion of concentration gradient.

Reading Assignment

Chap. 2, pp. 31–43.

Self-Test

Part I

Directions: Circle the correct answer(s).

1. When a system has reached diffusion equilibrium the following conditions exist.
   a Concentration on both sides of the membrane is equal.
   b The temperature of the system is decreased.
   c The net flux is zero.
   d Random movement of the molecules is decreased.

2. The force which drives bulk flow results from a difference in

   a pressure. *b* concentration.
   c osmolarity. *d* permeability.

3. Which of the following illustrate(s) bulk flow?

   a blood flow
   b exchange of molecules between a cell and its immediate environment
   c exchange of gases between the atmosphere and the lungs
   d exchange of gases between the lungs and the blood

Part II

Directions: Circle T for true and F for false.

T F 1. A flux of molecules occurs in both directions in a concentration gradient.
T F 2. The basic diffusion equation reflects the fact that net flux is related to the concentration between compartments.
T F 3. Bulk flow involves the random movement of molecules from one point to another.
T F 4. Movement of O_2 from the lungs to the blood is an example of bulk flow in the gaseous state.
T F 5. At diffusion equilibrium there is no movement of particles in either direction.

Part III

Directions: Complete the following items in the space provided.

1. Diffusion involves movement of material from a (higher/lower)

   ______________________ concentration to a

   (higher/lower) ______________________ concentration.
2. The amount of material which crosses a given boundary in a given amount of time is

   described as ______________________.

3. The magnitude of the flux is determined by the ______________________ gradient on the solution.

4. The equation for bulk flow is ______________________.
5. Net flux into a cell can be defined by the equation

   ______________________.

6. A high lipid solubility in a molecule is associated with a (large/small)

   ______________________ permeability constant.

7. The basic equation for diffusion is ______________________.

Module II: Mediated Transport and Osmosis

Objectives

Upon completion of this module, the student will be able to:

1. Describe the carrier hypothesis in mediated transport.
2. Define the terms *chemical specificity, competition,* and *saturation* in relation to the carrier hypothesis.
3. Define and differentiate between facilitated diffusion and active transport.
4. Define *pinocytosis* and *phagocytosis.*
5. Define and differentiate between molar concentration and osmolar concentration.
6. Define *osmosis.*
7. Define *isotonic, hypotonic,* and *hypertonic* solutions and their effects on cell volume.

Reading Assignment

Chap. 2, pp. 43–54.

Self-Test

Part I

Directions: Circle T for true and F for false.

T F 1. During mediated transport, a molecule binds to the membrane which facilitates its movement through the membrane.

T F 2. Mediated transport is a mechanism for moving lipid soluble molecules across cell membranes.

T F 3. The carrier molecule moves outside the membrane to pick up a solute molecule and carries it into the cell.

T F 4. In facilitated diffusion the carrier moves the molecules from a region of low concentration to one of high concentration.

Part II

Directions: Complete the following items in the space provided.

1. The term used to refer to the total concentration of all solute particles in solution is

   ______________________.
2. An important defense mechanism of the body is the ability of white blood cells to engulf

   bacteria by ______________________.
3. In pinocytosis the contents of the vesicle formed are

   ______________________. In phagocytosis they are

   ______________________.

4. If a membrane is impermeable to certain solutes then the movement of water as the result of a solute concentration difference is referred to as

 ________________________________.

5. A solution containing 0.3 osmoles per liter of a (penetrating/nonpenetrating) ________________________________ solute causes the cell to swell up.
6. When a membrane is transporting a substance at its maximum capacity it is said to be

 ________________________________.

7. The ability of mediated transport systems to identify and transport the correct chemical substance is known as ________________________________.
8. A cell will shrink when placed in a ________________________________ solution.
9. As the osmolarity of a solution increases the water concentration

 ________________________________.

10. The osmolarity of 1 mole of glucose in 1 liter of water is ________; of 1 mole of sodium chloride in 1 liter of water; ________; of 1 mole of glucose and 1 mole of sodium chloride in 1 liter of water; ________.

Part III

Directions: Fill in the blanks as indicated.

1. In the following list, label examples of bulk flow with B, diffusion with D, and mediated transports with M.

 a ________exchange of gases between the lungs and the blood

 b ________exchange of gases between the atmosphere and the lungs

 c ________movement of molecules with high lipid solubility into the cell

 d ________uptake of glucose by the cell

 e ________water movement across the cell membrane

 f ________uptake of amino acids by the cell

2. If a cell has an intracellular concentration of 0.3 osmolar, give the concentration or description of the following extracellular solutions or actions, using O for hypotonic, I for isotonic, and H for hypertonic.

 a ________0.5 osm *b* ________0.3 osm

 c ________causing the cell to shrink *d* ________0.2 osm

 e ________causing the cell to swell

3. Which of the following requires metabolic energy?

 a osmosis *b* diffusion

 c facilitated diffusion *d* active transport

4. According to the carrier hypothesis saturation can be explained by the fact that carrier molecules

   a move only in one direction.
   b operate cyclically, only a few being available at any given time.
   c are finite in number.

5. Competition is most likely to occur between which two of the following?

   a two different amino acids
   b an amino acid and a sugar
   c two different simple sugars
   d a protein and a sugar
   e a protein and a carbohydrate

Module III: Membrane Structure and Junctions

Objectives

Upon completion of this module the student will be able to:

1. Describe the polar and nonpolar molecules of the membrane and their location and function in membrane structure.
2. Describe the appearance of the cell membrane as seen with an electron microscope.
3. Describe the role of protein in the explanation of the permeability of membranes to ions like sodium, potassium, and chloride.
4. Describe the bimolecular organization of lipids in the cell membrane.
5. Describe and differentiate among a desmosome, a tight junction, and a gap junction and give an example of each.

Reading Assignment

Chap. 2, pp. 54–60.

Self-Test

Part I

Directions: Circle T for true and F for false.

T F 1. Cholesterol is the major lipid component of the cell membrane.
T F 2. Some proteins extend all the way through the membrane and are exposed on both sides.

T F 3. In forming a phospholipid bilayer the polar phosphate ends are attracted to one another.

T F 4. At a tight junction the cytoplasm of the two cells is linked by small channels.

T F 5. Gap junctions transmit electrical activity from one cell to another.

T F 6. The lipid portion of the membrane provides the major barrier to diffusion of molecules across the membrane.

Part II

Directions: Circle the correct answer(s).

1. Proteins passing all the way through the membrane provide channels for the passage of

   a lipids. *b* glucose. *c* ions. *d* amino acids.

2. The major structural components of membranes are

   a lipids. *b* carbohydrates. *c* proteins. *d* steroids.

Part III

Directions: Complete the following items in the space provided.

1. The uncharged portion of a phospholipid consists of

   ______________________________.

2. The three layers seen in the electron micrograph of cell membranes correspond in chemical composition to the outer layer of ______________________________, middle layer of ______________________________, and inner layer of ______________________________.

3. A junction commonly found in areas of mechanical stress is

   ______________________________.

4. The junction which blocks the diffusion of polar molecules across epithelial cell layers is a(n)

   ______________________________.

5. Which junction—D for desmosome, G for gap junction, T for tight junction—is most likely to be found in each of the following locations:

   a ________skin

   b ________smooth muscle

   c ________intestinal lining (as a diffusion barrier)

   d ________cardiac muscle (for communication)

   e ________cardiac muscle (for stress)

Module I:
Energy, Chemical Reactions, and Enzymes

Module II:
ATP and Metabolic Pathways

ENERGY AND CELLULAR METABOLISM

CHAPTER 3

Module I: Energy, Chemical Reactions, and Enzymes

Objectives

Upon completion of this module, the student will be able to:

1. Define *metabolism, catabolic reactions, anabolic reactions, dynamic equilibrium, energy, calorie, activation energy, enzyme, coenzyme,* and *vitamin.*
2. Describe and give examples of the law of mass action.
3. Specify the effect of temperature on the rate of chemical reactions.
4. Describe the mechanism of enzyme action, including the concept of active site and chemical specificity.
5. List the three major factors influencing the rate of enzyme-mediated reactions as concentration of substrate, concentration of enzymes, and the activity of individual enzyme molecules.
6. Define *enzyme induction, enzyme repression,* and *modulator molecule.*
7. Describe the difference between reversible and irreversible chemical reactions.
8. Describe the role of rate-limiting enzymes in metabolic pathways.

Reading Assignment

Chap. 3, pp. 61–72.

Self-Test

Part I

Directions: Match the words in column A with their definitions from column B. Place the letter of the definition in column B in the blank preceding the word to be defined in column A.

Column A	Column B
1. ______ metabolism	*a* amount of heat energy needed to raise temperature of 1 gram H_2O by 1°C
2. ______ catabolic reaction	*b* a protein catalyst
3. ______ anabolic reaction	*c* total collection of chemical reactions occurring within a living organism
4. ______ energy	*d* puts small molecule fragments together to form larger molecules (synthesis)
5. ______ activation energy	*e* ability to perform work
6. ______ dynamic equilibrium	*f* results in fragmentation (breakdown) of molecule

7. ________ coenzyme
8. ________ calorie
9. ________ enzyme

g low-molecular-weight substance required for the activity of certain enzymes (often vitamin derivatives)
h energy required to initiate a chemical reaction
i rates of synthesis = rate of degradation

Part II

Directions: Answer each of the questions below in the space provided.

1. Describe the law of mass action.

2. Describe the concept of activation energy.

3. Describe how the activity of an enzyme can be altered.

4. Write a formula for the reaction between an enzyme and a substrate.

Part III

Directions: Circle the correct answer(s).

1. Rates of chemical reactions vary with

   a temperature.
   b magnitude of activation energy.
   c concentration of enzymes.
   d concentration of reactants.
   e activity of enzyme molecules.

2. Which of the following are examples of the law of mass action when considering the reaction

   $A + B \rightleftharpoons X + Y$ A, B, X, Y are all equal concentrations at equilibrium

   a Addition of *A* causes an increase in *X* and *Y*.
   b Addition of *A* causes an increase in *X*, but does not affect the concentration of *Y*.
   c Addition of *A* increases the concentration of *A*, *B*, *X*, and *Y*.
   d Addition of *A* results in a reduction of the concentration of *B*.
   e Addition of *A* will affect only the concentration of *A*.

3. Adding heat to a chemical reaction
   a increases the kinetic energy of molecules.
   b increases the rate of molecular motion.
   c slows down molecules so they react better.
   d increases the frequency of molecular collisions.
4. In altering enzymatic activity, modulators
   a bind with the enzyme active site.
   b change the shape of the active site.
   c bind with the enzyme at a location other than the active site.
   d always increase the activity of the enzyme.

Module II: ATP and Metabolic Pathways

Objectives

Upon completion of this module, the student will be able to:

1. Describe the role of ATP in cellular metabolism.
2. Define *glycolysis, oxidative phosphorylation, Krebs cycle, anaerobic glycolysis.*
3. Identify the location of the enzymes involved in oxidative phosphorylation, and specify the end products.
4. Identify the location of enzymes and the end products of aerobic and anaerobic glycolysis.
5. Diagram the relation between glycolysis, the Krebs cycle, and oxidative phosphorylation (as shown in Fig. 3-21, p. 84).
6. Identify the amount of ATP that is formed during the metabolism of one mole of glucose by anaerobic glycolysis and by aerobic metabolism.
7. Describe the chemical structure and function of glycogen.
8. Identify the common products of glucose and fatty acid metabolism which enter mitochondrial oxidative metabolism to produce CO_2, ATP, H_2O, and heat (see Fig. 3-24, p. 86).
9. Compare the amount of ATP produced from the oxidative metabolism of 1 gram of glucose with 1 gram of triglyceride.
10. Identify the nitrogen-containing end product of protein metabolism.
11. Describe the possible and impossible interconversion of carbohydrates, fats, and proteins.
12. Describe the energy cycle linking sunlight and photosynthesis in plants with oxidative metabolism in animals.

Reading Assignment

Chap. 3, pp. 72–89.

Self-Test

Part I

Directions: Complete the following items in the space provided.

1. Most ATP synthesis within cells occurs in the ________________________________,

   by the process of ________________________________.
2. What is the energy yield of 1 g of triglyceride? of glucose?

3. During oxidative phosphorylation, molecular oxygen combines with

   ________________________________ to produce

   ________________________________. The energy released in this reaction is used to

   form ________________________________.
4. Carbon dioxide is formed during the chemical reactions known as

   ________________________________ which occur in the

   ________________________________.

Part II

Directions; Circle the correct answer(s).

1. Oxidative phosphorylation

   a permits an efficient recovery of energy.
   b cannot proceed without oxygen.
   c takes place in the mitochondria.
   d permits approximately a 40 percent energy recovery.
   e regenerates the coenzyme NAD for another cycle.
2. Anaerobic glycolysis

   a occurs in the absence of oxygen.
   b results in a net gain of 4 ATP/mole of glucose.
   c leads to the formation of lactic acid as its end product.
   d occurs in the mitochondria of the cell.
3. Concerning the interconversion of carbohydrate, lipid, and protein—

   a all three classes can enter the Krebs cycle through some intermediate.
   b glucose can be converted into fat or amino acids.
   c fatty acids can be converted into glucose.
   d amino acids can be converted to fat.
   e all amino acids can be converted to glucose by a process called oxidative deamination.

Part III

Directions: Circle T for true and F for false.

T F 1. The end product of anaerobic glycolysis is lactic acid.

T F 2. Most of the glucose in food is either broken down to yield energy or is stored as glycogen.

T F 3. Glycogen is stored primarily in the muscles and the liver.

T F 4. The breakdown of glucose produces acetyl CoA, the main ingredient for fatty acid synthesis.

T F 5. The oxygen used by animals (for the release of energy from glucose) originated from plants by photosynthesis.

Module I:
Genetics

Module II:
Development

PROTEIN SYNTHESIS, HEREDITY, AND CELL DEVELOPMENT

CHAPTER 4

Module I: Genetics

Objectives

Upon completion of this module, the student will be able to:

1. Define *DNA, RNA, chromosome, double helix, base pairing, gene, codon, nucleotide, base,* and *ribosome.*
2. Explain why controlling protein synthesis is crucial to controlling a cell's structure and function.
3. State the differences between DNA and RNA.
4. Describe the three-base sequence of the genetic code used for specifying the location of amino acids in a protein.
5. Describe the synthesis of messenger RNA (mRNA) from DNA.
6. Define *ribosomal RNA* (rRNA) and *transfer RNA* (tRNA).
7. Describe the interaction of mRNA, ribosomes, and tRNA in protein assembly.
8. Define *polyribosomes, secretory granules, lysosomes.*
9. State the role of the endoplasmic reticulum and the Golgi apparatus in protein secretion.
10. List four sites at which regulation of protein synthesis could occur.
11. Describe induction and repression; differentiate between repression and end-product inhibition.
12. Describe the control of mRNA synthesis in terms of the operon, repressor protein, operator gene, and inducing molecule.

Reading Assignment

Chap. 4, pp. 90–111.

Self-Test

Part I

Directions: Match the items in column A with those in column B. Each item in column A may have more than one match, and items in column B may be used more than once.

Column A	Column B
1. ________ usually carry the information required to synthesize a single protein or molecule of RNA	*a* gene
2. ________ a single molecule of DNA may include many of these	*b* RNA
3. ________ the largest molecules in the cell	*c* DNA
4. ________ the chemical subunits of nucleic acids	*d* nucleotide
5. ________ consists of three component parts	*e* chromosome
	f base
	g nucleolus
	h codon

6. ________ transmits hereditary characteristics from cell to cell
7. ________ nitrogen-containing part of nucleic acid
8. ________ chemically differentiates the nucleic acids from one another
9. ________ three-base sequence for single amino acid

Part II

Directions: Circle the correct answer(s).

1. Ribonucleic acid (RNA)

   a is the basic carrier of genetic information from cell to cell.
   b is a protein.
   c is composed of the same nucleotides found in DNA.
   d transfers information from DNA in the nucleus to the site of protein synthesis.

2. Most protein synthesis occurs in the

   a nucleus. *b* nucleolus.
   c cytoplasm. *d* mitochondria.
   e extracellular fluid.

3. Which of the following identify *differences* between DNA and RNA?

   a number of strands in a molecule
   b base composition
   c sugar composition
   d number of different bases in a single molecule
   e types of chemical linkage between bases
   f rate of synthesis and degradation of the average molecule

4. The genetic code for DNA includes which of the following?

   a base sequences forming nonsense codons
   b only four bases
   c codons composed of base sequences
   d variable codon size
   e gene codon sequences of varying length
   f four bases designating one codon
   g potentially 64 codons
   h three base codons, *each* of which corresponds to an amino acid, different codons
   i is degenerate; i.e., different codons describe the same amino acid

5. Which of the following is (are) true of messenger RNA?

   a When DNA unwinds in the synthesis of mRNA, only one of the two DNA chains is used to form a single mirror-image chain of mRNA.
   b The formation of mRNA does *not* involve making a mirror-image of the entire DNA molecule.

c DNA codon C-G-T becomes mRNA codon G-C-A.
d DNA codon G-C-A becomes mRNA codon C-G-T.

6. Choose the proper order for the following sequence of events leading from DNA to protein synthesis.

   (1) Elongation of protein chain.
   (2) mRNA passes from the nucleus to the cytoplasm where one end of the mRNA molecule binds to a ribosome.
   (3) Free amino acids combine with their corresponding tRNAs.
   (4) Transcription of DNA to mRNA.
   (5) The three base anticodons in tRNA pair with the corresponding codons in mRNA attached to the ribosomes.
   (6) Termination of protein chain.

   a 1, 2, 3, 4, 5, 6 *b* 4, 6, 2, 1, 3, 5
   c 3, 6, 2, 5, 1, 4 *d* 2, 5, 4, 6, 1, 3
   e 4, 2, 3, 5, 1, 6

7. Which of the following are correct?

   a In enzyme repression, the synthesis of a series of enzymes is prevented.
   b In enzyme end-product inhibition, the activity of an enzyme that has already been synthesized is reduced.
   c In enzyme induction, the synthesis of a series of enzymes is increased.

8. The control of mRNA synthesis is achieved by a repression-induction process. Which of the following form a part of this control?

   a A repressor *gene* contains the coded information for the synthesis of a repressor protein
   b A repressor *protein* is synthesized in the standard way via a repressor gene.
   c The repressor protein may combine with the initial gene of an operon, known as the *operator* gene.
   d The repressor gene is part of a DNA molecule.
   e The combination of the repressor *protein* with the operator gene prevents synthesis of of the operon's mRNA.
   f The induction process occurs when an *inducer molecule* combines with the repressor protein, thereby inactivating the repressor.

Part III

Directions: Complete the following items in the space provided.

1. A type of cell organelle which is a vesicular body containing a variety of very potent digestive enzymes capable of chopping up almost any molecule with which it comes into contact is called a(n) ________________________.
2. A number of ribosomes attached to the same strand of mRNA form what is known as a(n) ________________________.
3. The vesicles which cells use to package and externalize the proteins that have been synthesized and released to the cytoplasm by the Golgi apparatus are called ________________________.

4. List four sites at which regulation of protein synthesis could occur.

a ____________________

b ____________________

c ____________________

d ____________________

Module II: **Development**

Objectives

Upon completion of this module, the student will be able to:

1. Distinguish among cell growth, replication, and differentiation.
2. Describe the process of DNA replication in terms of DNA separation, template formation, and complementary strand production.
3. Describe the process of cell division, using the terms chromosome, chromatin, interphase, centromere, spindle apparatus, and centriole.
4. Differentiate between mitosis and meiosis.
5. Define *mutation.*
6. List environmental factors which increase the rate of mutations.
7. Define *natural selection* and describe the process by which it occurs.
8. Describe a virus and its method of replication.
9. State the major abnormality of cancer.

Reading Assignment

Chap. 4, pp. 111–118.

Self-Test

Part I

Directions: Circle the letter of the correct answer(s).

1. The process of a DNA molecule splitting, and the pairing of free nucleotides with the bases of each DNA strand to give rise to two new molecules of DNA, each containing one new and one old strand, is best named

   a transcription. *b* reverse transcription.
   c replication. *d* duplication.
   e differentiation.

2. Which of the following statements are true concerning the process of cell division?

   a Most cells spend most of their time in the interphase period of cell division.
   b During *early* cell division, when DNA threads have been duplicated, they are joined together over a small segment of their length in a region known as the centriole.
   c The combination of nucleic acid and protein forms a nucleoprotein known as a centromere.
   d The process of cell division in nonreproductive cells is called mitosis.
   e The spindle fibers of the spindle apparatus act as if they are pulling the chromosome segments toward the poles of the cell during division.

3. Which of the following is (are) true regarding meiosis? It

   a involves the reproductive cells.
   b results in four daughter cells containing 23 chromosomes each.
   c often leads to exchange of genetic information between maternal and paternal chromosomes.
   d involves a series of four cell divisions in succession.

4. Which of the following are major environmental factors which increase the rate of mutations?

   a atomic radiation *b* sunlight *c* x-rays
   d moonlight *e* cosmic rays *f* certain chemicals
   g ultraviolet light *h* reading physiology texts

5. Which of the following are true of natural selection?

   a is not affected by mutations
   b may result in a sturdier, more effective organism
   c may result in a weaker, less effective organism
   d occurs slowly, over long periods of time
   e has no effect on survival rates of organisms
   f small changes that are beneficial (given enough time) can produce large changes in the structure and function of an organism

6. Which of the following are true of a virus?

   a contains all the normal components of a cell
   b metabolizes in the normal way
   c cannot reproduce by itself
   d consists only of a molecule of nucleic acid surrounded by several molecules of protein
   e can provide its own energy for duplication
   f may have either DNA or RNA as its nucleic acid for reproduction

Module I:
Internal Environment

Module II:
Control Systems

Module III:
Balance Concept and Biological Rhythms

THE INTERNAL ENVIRONMENT AND HOMEOSTASIS

CHAPTER 5

Module I: Internal Environment

Objectives

Upon completion of this module, the student will be able to:

1. Differentiate between chemical and biological evolution and describe the significance of proteinoids in the development of unicellular organisms.
2. Define *internal environment* in terms of the cell membrane and extracellular fluid.
3. Differentiate between interstitial fluid and extracellular fluid.
4. List and give the percentage for each component of total body water.
5. Identify the differences in ionic composition of intracellular and extracellular fluid and state the reason why these differences can exist.
6. Define *homeostasis*.
7. Name the two intracellular communication systems.

Reading Assignment

Chap. 5, pp. 120–124.

Exercises

Part I

Some ion concentrations are characteristically higher on one side of a membrane than on the other. On the basis of the ions shown, label each side as intracellular or extracellular.

K^+ Mg^+ Cl^- Na^+

1. ______________________ 2. ______________________ (*123*)

Part II

Evolution occurring over millions of years may have passed through some of the following stages. Label each as biological or chemical evolution.

aerobic animal organisms 1. ______________________

↑

unicellular organisms 2. ______________________

↑

DNA, RNA 3. ______________________

↑

polypeptides 4. ______________________

↑

simple organic molecules 5. ______________________ (*121*)

Part III

Water is an important component of the body and makes up a large portion of the body weight. Determine the weight of each of the following fluid components in a 150-lb person.

1. intracellular fluid ______________________
2. extracellular fluid ______________________
3. interstitial fluid ______________________
4. plasma ______________________ (*123*)

Self-Test

Part I

Directions: Circle T for true and F for false.

T F 1. The cell membrane is unaffected by the fluid surrounding it.
T F 2. Intracellular fluid makes up a larger part of total body water than does extracellular fluid.
T F 3. The cell interior has ionic concentrations similar to those of extracellular fluid.

Part II

Directions: Complete each of the following items in the space provided.

1. Fluctuations in the internal environment are kept to a minimum by regulatory responses. The stable condition which results is known as ______________________.
2. The chance formation of organic molecules was an important step in ______________________.
3. The most striking parallel between extracellular fluid and sea water is a high concentration of ______________________.
4. Polypeptides, when treated with hot water, separate out as membrane-bound microspheres called ______________________.
5. Extracellular fluid is divided between two compartments. They are ______________________ and ______________________.

Part III

Directions: Indicate whether the concentration of each of the following ions is characteristically higher in intracellular or extracellular fluid.

_______ K^+

_______ Cl^-

_______ Na^+

_______ Mg^+

A. intracellular fluid
B. extracellular fluid

Module II: Control Systems

Objectives

Upon completion of this module, the student will be able to:

1. Define *homeostatic* or *control systems.*
2. Differentiate between steady-state condition and the maintenance of a precise set point.
3. Describe a negative feedback system in terms of its ability to regulate a variable around the initial value rather than preventing an initial displacement (see Fig. 5-5, p. 125).
4. Diagram a reflex arc including the five components of the system as well as the stimulus, response, and feedback.
5. Differentiate between a homeostatic reflex and a local homeostatic response.
6. Define *receptor site* and differentiate it from a receptor in a reflex arc.
7. Define *chemical mediator.*

Reading Assignment

Chap. 5, pp. 124–130. Note particularly Fig. 5-6, p. 126.

Exercises

Part I

Directions: Complete the following items in the space provided.

A moderate blow to the jaw results in flexing of the jaw-opening muscles. This is known as the jaw jerk reflex.

1. What is the stimulus for this reflex? ______________________________
2. What is the general term for the structure which detects the stimulus?

   ____

3. Indicate the response in this reflex. ______________________________
4. Identify each of the numbers in Fig. W-2, which is a line diagram of a reflex.

(1) ______________________________ (2) ______________________________

(3) ______________________________ (4) ______________________________

(126–127)

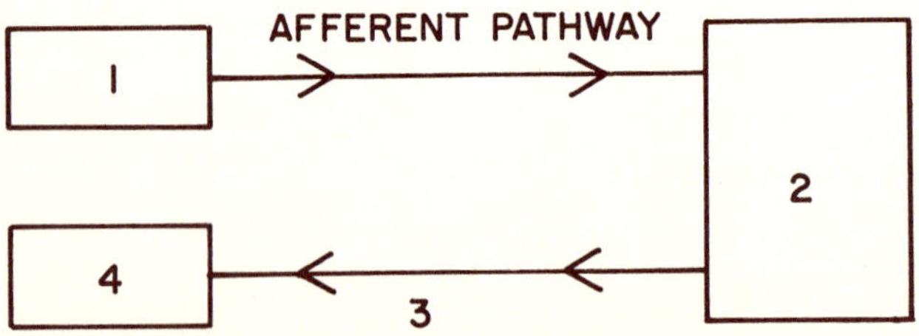

Fig. W-2

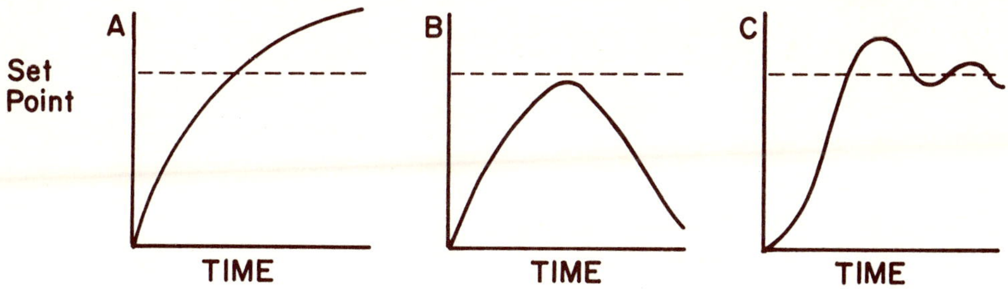

Fig. W-3

Part II

Which of the graphs in Fig. W-3 illustrates a system maintained by negative feedback control? Explain. *(125–126)*

Self-Test

Part I

Directions: Circle T for true and F for false.

T F 1. Negative feedback is effective for preventing any change from a precise set point.
T F 2. A local homeostatic response involves neither hormones nor nerves.
T F 3. For maintenance of blood calcium levels, the parathyroid glands act as the effector. (See Fig. 5-8, p. 128.)

Part II

Directions: Circle the correct answer(s).

1. A receptor site is

   a the same for all types of chemical mediators.
   b generally within the cell membrane structure of many cells.
   c that portion of the reflex arc which detects environmental changes.

2. Negative feedback systems

   a can anticipate a pending change in the system.
   b react explosively to cause further disturbance.
   c restore the regulated variable around normal.
   d increase the instability of the system.

3. An afferent receptor

   a is the same as a membrane receptor site.
   b detects the stimulus in a reflex.
   c is generally formed by bone or muscle.
   d always makes an individual aware of the stimulus.

4. The efferent pathway
   a can be a hormone.
   b transmits information from an effector to the integrating center.
   c is connected directly to the receptor.
   d can be a nerve.

Module III: Balance Concept and Biological Rhythms

Objectives

Upon completion of this module, the student will be able to:

1. Describe the balance concept in terms of pool, net gain, net loss, and distribution.
2. Diagram the essential elements involved in the balance concept as depicted in Fig. 5-9, p. 130.
3. List the three possible states that can occur in total body balance and indicate how each state comes about.
4. Describe the two criteria necessary for a substance to be considered an essential nutrient.
5. Describe the relative or absolute nature of chemical homeostasis.
6. Differentiate between the minimal and optimal intake of a nutrient.
7. Differentiate between general biological rhythms and circadian rhythms.

Reading Assignment

Chap. 5, pp. 130–132. Note particularly Fig. 5-9, p. 130.

Exercises

1. Label the elements of the balance concept which are depicted by number in Fig. W-4.

   (1) ______________________ (2) ______________________

   (3) ______________________ (4) ______________________

2. Three states of body balance are possible. What are they and how do they relate to (1) and (2) above? *(130–131)*

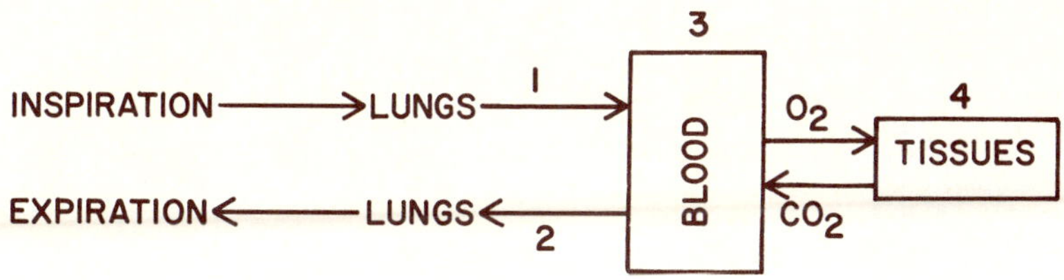

Fig. W-4

Self-Test

Part I

Directions: Circle the correct answer(s).

1. The term circadian rhythms refers to events which occur

   a daily. *b* every other day.
   c weekly. *d* monthly.

2. To be considered essential a nutrient must be

   a found in the diet.
   b necessary for survival.
   c synthesized in inadequate amounts in the body.
   d synthesized in large amounts in the body.
   e necessary for blood formation.

3. Which of the following are essential nutrients?

   a glucose *b* meat *c* water

Part II

Directions: Complete the following items in the space provided.

1. When the body's net gain is greater than its net loss, this is known as

   ______________________________.

2. One of the best-known examples of a general biological rhythm is

   ______________________________.

3. The state of total body balance is dependent on both elements of the balance concept. These

   are ______________________________ and

   ______________________________.

Part III

Directions: Circle T for true and F for false.

T F 1. Homeostatic responses are able to hold the internal environment absolutely constant.
T F 2. Optimal intake is the same for differing factors and situations.
T F 3. Positive balance occurs when net gain is greater than net loss.

Module I:
Electrical Properties of the Neuron, Part I

Module II:
Electrical Properties of the Neuron, Part II

Module III:
Electrical Properties of the Neuron, Part III

Module IV:
Functional Anatomy of Neurons

Module V:
Synapses

Module VI:
Divisions of the Nervous System

CHAPTER 6 NEURAL CONTROL MECHANISMS

Module I: Electrical Properties of the Neuron, Part I

Objectives

Upon completion of this module, the student will be able to:

1. State the nature of the force acting between two similar and two different electrical charges (i.e., attraction or repulsion).
2. Describe, using the equation $W = f(x)$, how work must be done or energy released when the distance between two charged particles is increased or decreased.
3. Define *voltage* and *potential difference* and describe their relation to volt and millivolt.
4. Define *insulator* and *conductor* and give examples of each in biological systems.
5. Define *current* and *resistance* and describe their relationships to voltage and potential difference.
6. Define *membrane potential,* how and where it is measured, and the range and orientation of this potential.
7. Define and differentiate between *diffusion potential* and *equilibrium potential.*
8. State the relationships between active transport, membrane permeability, and concentration gradients.
9. Define *resting membrane potential* and describe its magnitude, direction, concentration gradients involved, and its maintenance.

Reading Assignment

Chap. 6, pp. 133–140.

Exercises

Part I

Directions: Answer the following questions, which refer to Fig. W-5, in the space provided.

1. As the situation changes from A to B, is work done?

   ____

   Is energy released? ____________________

2. As the situation changes from B to A, is work done?

   ____

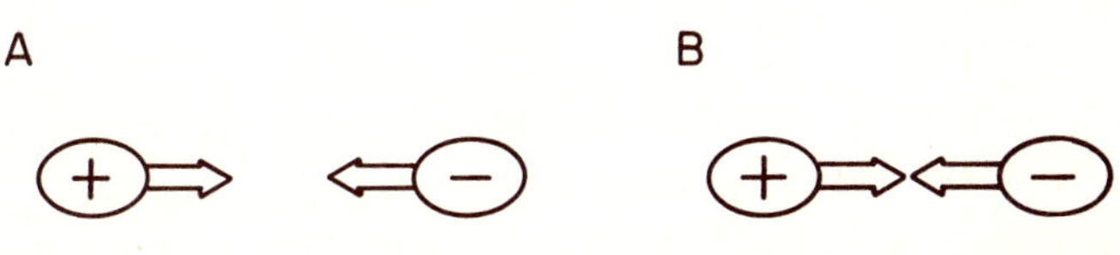

Fig. W-5

What can you say about the energy? ____________________

____

3. In which case is the force between the particles greater, A or B?

____

4. Write the equation for work which describes these relationships.

____________________ (*134–135*)

Part II

Directions: Answer the following questions in the space provided.

1. On the basis of charge, label the sides of Fig. W-6 as intracellular or extracellular.

   (1) ____________________

   (2) ____________________

2. What ions are referred to in the diagram?

   (3) ____________________

   (4) ____________________

3. What is the "structure" labeled (5)? Explain its role in the maintenance of the membrane potential. (*139*)

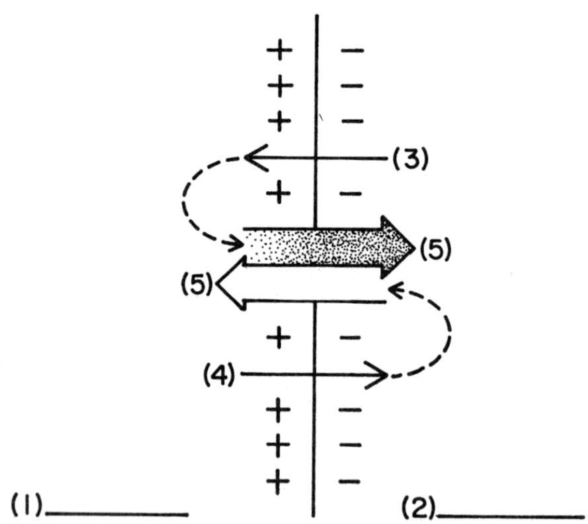

Fig. W-6

Self-Test

Part I

Directions: Circle T for true and F for false.

T F 1. The magnitude of the resting membrane potential varies from 5 to 10 mV depending on the type of cell.
T F 2. The inside of the cell is negatively charged with respect to the outside.
T F 3. Sodium and chloride ions which have diffused into the cell are actively transported back out of the cell.
T F 4. The extracellular water compartments in the body act as good insulators for the cells.
T F 5. The units of measurement of potential difference are volts.
T F 6. The cell membrane is more permeable to sodium than to potassium.

Part II

Directions: Circle the correct answer(s).

1. The movement of electric charge is known as

   a voltage. *b* resistance.
   c current. *d* potential.

2. Which of the following ions shows no net diffusion across the resting membrane?

   a sodium *b* potassium *c* chloride

3. In the equation for work, $W = F(x)$, x equals

   a the charge on the particles.
   b the distance through which the force acts.
   c the potential difference between the starting and finishing points.

4. As two unlike charges move farther apart,

   a work must be done on the particles.
   b the particles themselves are doing work.
   c energy is released from the system.
   d energy must be put into the system.

Module II: Electrical Properties of the Neuron, Part II

Objectives

Upon completion of this module, the student will be able to:

1. Define and diagram the terms *depolarize, hyperpolarize,* and *repolarize* (see Fig. 6-11, p. 140).
2. Define *action potential* and describe the change in membrane permeability, ion net fluxes, and ionic activation and inactivation that take place during the action potential.
3. Describe and diagram the positive feedback relationship in sodium activation (see Fig. 6-13, p. 142).
4. Define *threshold potential* and differentiate between threshold and resting membrane potential.
5. Define *threshold stimulus* and *excitability.*
6. Define and differentiate between *subthreshold* and *suprathreshold stimulus.*

Reading Assignment

Chap. 6, pp. 140–143.

Exercises

Directions: Answer the following questions in the space provided.

A nerve fiber is given a suprathreshold stimulus.

1. What is the first major change in the membrane? (*141*)

2. In the space below, diagram the positive-feedback mechanism of this sodium permeability change. (*142*)

3. What are the mechanisms that bring the membrane back to a resting potential? (*141*)

4. The property of excitability is found in two types of cells. This property makes

_______________ and

_______________ cells capable of producing

_______________. (*140*)

Self-Test

Part I

Directions: Circle T for true, and F for false.

T F 1. The critical level to which the membrane must be depolarized to trigger an action potential is known as the threshold potential.
T F 2. As the membrane potential moves closer to threshold, it becomes hyperpolarized.
T F 3. An action potential results from a transient change in concentration gradients.
T F 4. Sodium activation refers to an increase in sodium permeability.
T F 5. Threshold potential is further from zero than the resting membrane potential.

Part II

Directions: Complete the following items in the space provided.

1. The property of nerve and muscle cells which makes them capable of producing action potentials is known as _______________.
2. A stimulus to a nerve or muscle cell which does not reach threshold is termed _______________.
3. In the initial stages of the action potential, the permeability of the membrane to sodium increases _______________-fold.
4. During an action potential, sodium permeability, after rising to its peak, is rapidly turned off. This is termed _______________.
5. Once a threshold level has been reached, the action potential that results is described as a(n) _______________ response.

Module III: Electrical Properties of the Neuron, Part III

Objectives

Upon completion of this module, the student will be able to:

1. Define *refractory period* and differentiate between absolute and relative refractory periods.
2. Describe the propagation of an action potential and differentiate this process from decremental conduction.
3. Describe what determines the direction of action potential propagation.
4. Describe the effect of myelin and fiber diameter on the velocity of action potential propagation.
5. Define *saltatory conduction.*

Reading Assignment

Chap. 6, pp. 144–146.

Exercises

Directions: Figure W-7 is a diagram of a myelinated nerve. Answer the following questions in the space provided.

1. What kind of conduction is illustrated? (*146*)

___

2. Is the speed of conduction in this neuron different from what it is in an unmyelinated nerve? Why? (*146*)

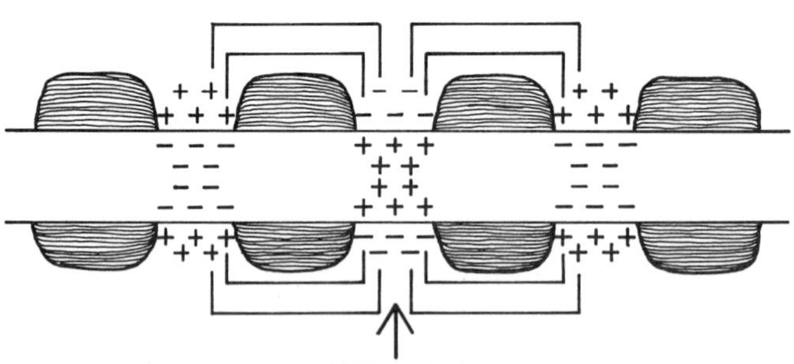

Fig. W-7

3. If the fiber is stimulated as indicated, put heads on the arrows to indicate the direction of ion flow. In which direction will the action potential travel? *(146–147)*

____

4. Define refractory period and explain its role in determining the direction of action potential propagation. *(144, 146)*

Self-Test

Part I

Directions: Circle T for true and F for false.

T F 1. During the absolute refractory period, the membrane cannot be stimulated.

T F 2. Saltatory conduction refers to the smooth, rapid movement of an action potential along an unmyelinated nerve.

T F 3. Because of the refractory period, action potentials move only away from the site of stimulation.

T F 4. The absolute refractory period corresponds to the period of sodium permeability changes.

T F 5. Action potential propagation is decremental.

Part II

Directions: Circle the correct answer(s).

1. The speed at which an action potential is transmitted depends on

   a fiber diameter.
   b fiber length.
   c whether or not the fiber is myelinated.
   d the number of branches along the membrane.

2. The relative refractory period corresponds to

   a decreased potassium permeability.
   b increased potassium permeability.
   c sodium permeability changes.
   d threshold potential which is further from zero.
   e threshold potential which is closer to zero.

3. A myelinated nerve is associated with

   a saltatory conduction.
   b decreased local current flow.
   c slower action potential conduction.

Module IV: Functional Anatomy of Neurons

Objectives

Upon completion of this module, the student will be able to:

1. Differentiate between the peripheral and central nervous system.
2. Describe a neuron, including axon, dendrite, initial segment, collaterals, and axon terminals.
3. Define and differentiate between afferent and efferent neurons.
4. Define and identify the location of interneurons.
5. State the three normal ways action potentials are initiated.
6. Define *receptor* and state its relation to afferent neurons and generator potentials.
7. List the differences between the generator potential and an action potential (see Table 6-2).
8. Describe summation of generator potentials.
9. Define *adaptation* and list three possible reasons for its occurrence.
10. Describe the relation between the amplitude of a generator potential and the frequency and size of action potentials.
11. Define *intensity coding* and describe two mechanisms which account for its occurrence.

Reading Assignment

Chap. 6, pp. 147–153.

Exercises

Part I

Directions: Answer the following questions in the space provided.

Label the two major divisions of the nervous system as shown in Fig. W-8.

(*a*) ______________________________

(*b*) ______________________________

List the three types of neurons shown. (*149*)

(*c*) ______________________________

(*d*) ______________________________

(*e*) ______________________________

Part II

Directions: Answer the following questions in the space provided.

Label the structures indicated on the diagram (Fig. W-9) of a neuron and its myelin sheath. (*147–149*)

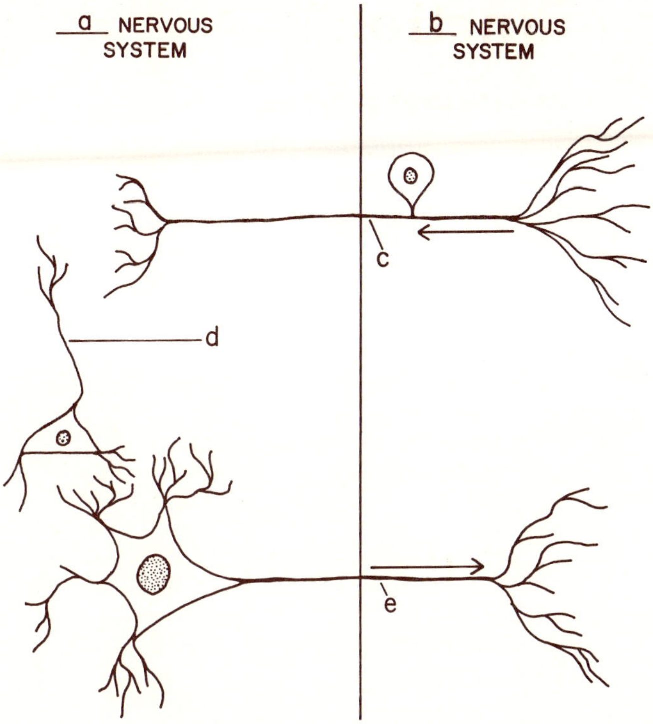

Fig. W-8

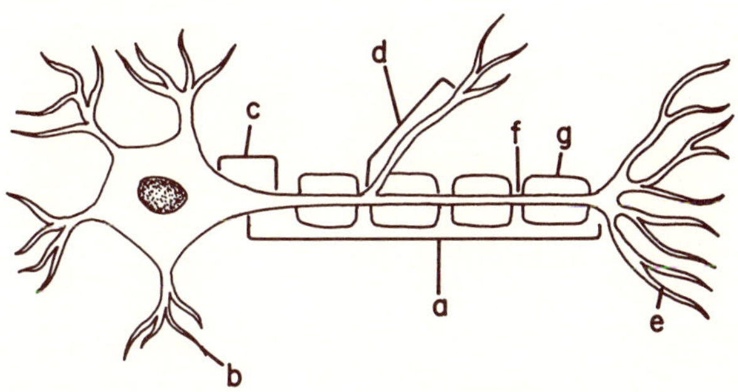

Fig. W-9

(a) ____________________

(b) ____________________

(c) ____________________

(d) ____________________

(e) ____________________

(f) ____________________

(g) ____________________

Self-Test

Part I

Directions: Complete the following items in the space provided.

1. As the amplitude of a generator potential increases, the size of the resultant action potential is

   ______________________.

2. A device which can accept selected energy forms and translate them into action potentials is known as a(n) ______________________.

3. As the amplitude of a generator potential increases, the resultant action potentials increase in

   ______________________.

4. Decrease in frequency of action potentials in afferent neurons despite constant stimulus is referred to as ____________ ____________.

5. In contrast to light touch, pressing the finger down hard on the skin stimulates additional receptors in a process known as ______________________.

Part II

Directions: Circle T for true, and F for false.

T F 1. Generator potentials are all or none.
T F 2. Interneurons are located only in the CNS.
T F 3. As the stimulus strength increases, the generator potentials increase in number but not in size.
T F 4. A generator potential has a refractory period slightly longer than that for an action potential.
T F 5. A node of Ranvier is an interruption in the myelin coating.

Part III

Directions: Circle the correct answer(s).

1. A generator potential is differentiated from an action potential because a generator potential
   a has a refractory period greater than 2 msec.
   b cannot be summed.
   c is a graded response.
   d travels by decremental conduction.

2. An action potential is differentiated from a generator potential because an action potential
   a has about a 1-msec refractory period.
   b cannot be summed.
   c has a duration greater than 2 msec.
   d has an amplitude which varies with the stimulus.

3. Which of the following is (are) true regarding receptors?
   a Most can be stimulated by different types of energy.
   b They react to different types of energy equally.
   c They communicate only with afferent and efferent neurons.
   d They are necessary for the reception of many energy forms.

Module V: Synapses

Objectives

Upon completion of this module, the student will be able to:

1. Differentiate between presynaptic and postsynaptic neurons.
2. Describe a synapse, including the concepts of synaptic cleft, synaptic vesicle, synaptic knob, subsynaptic membrane, and synaptic delay.
3. Differentiate between convergence and divergence as anatomical relationships between neurons.
4. Differentiate between excitatory and inhibitory synapses and their effect on the resting membrane potential.
5. Define *facilitation.*
6. Differentiate between spatial and temporal summation and describe their relationship to inhibition or excitation of a neuron.
7. Describe the significance of the lower threshold of the initial segment.
8. Describe how a postsynaptic cell functions as an integrator, using the concepts from objectives 3 to 7.
9. List five substances which appear to be chemical transmitters at synapses.
10. State the reason why synapses with chemical transmitters can conduct in only one direction.
11. Differentiate between an IPSP and presynaptic inhibition.
12. Differentiate between a neuroeffector transmitter and a synaptic transmitter. Give examples of each.
13. List the anatomic components of a reflex and describe the role of each in a simple reflex.

Reading Assignment

Chap. 6, pp. 154–162.

Exercises

Part I

Directions: Answer the following questions in the space provided.

1. In Fig. W-10, in which direction does the impulse flow?

   Describe the events occurring at the synapse to explain why this is so.

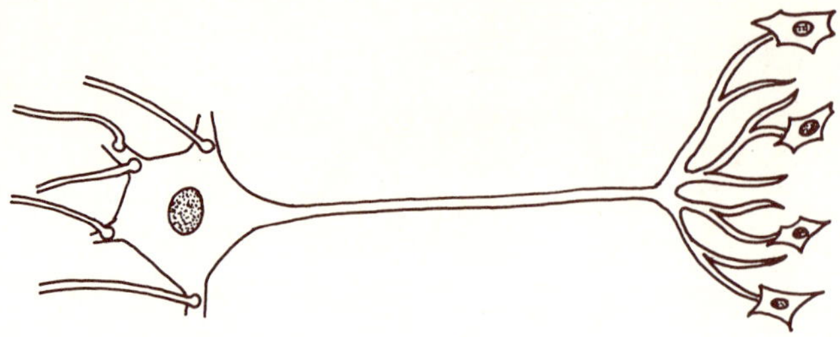

Fig. W-10

2. What is the term used to describe the relationship of the terminals on the left with the cell body they contact? ______________________
What term describes the branching of the center cell to affect many cells on the right?
____

3. There is a delay at the synapse of about 0.001 seconds in membrane changes by the post-synaptic cell. What is its cause?

Once the transmitter is released, describe three ways its effects on the postsynaptic cell can be terminated. *(154–156)*

Part II

Directions: Use the spaces provided to describe each part of the synapse shown in Fig. W-11.

A. ______________________ B. ______________________

C. ______________________ D. ______________________

E. ______________________ F. ______________________

Describe what the ion movement and resulting change in membrane potential would be if this were an inhibitory synapse. *(156)*

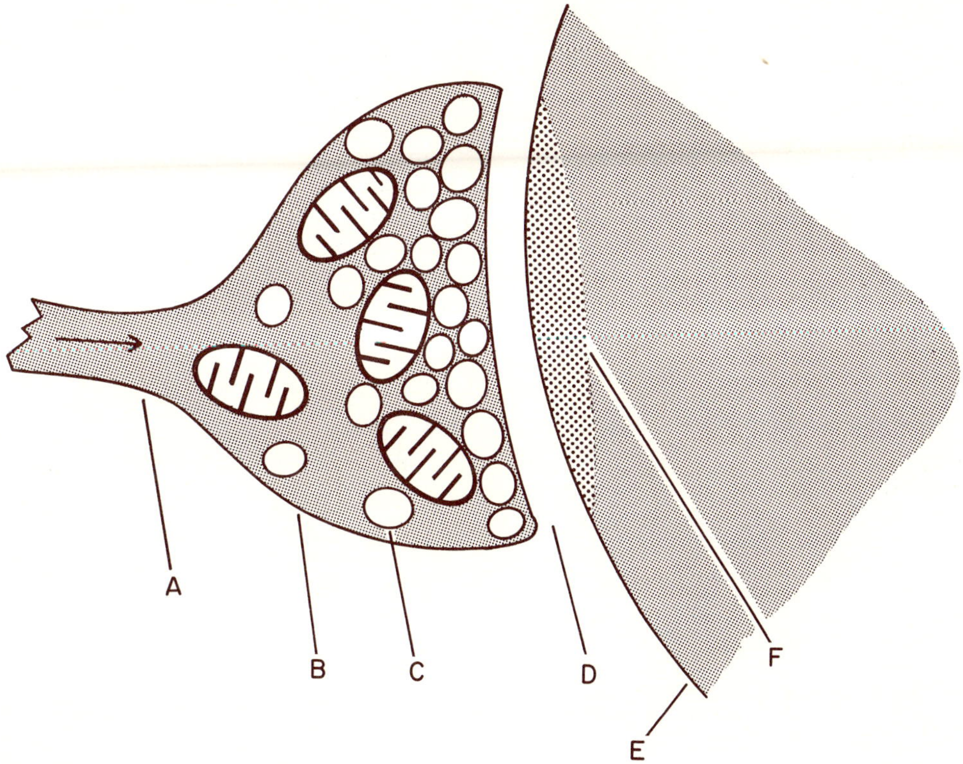

Fig. W-11

Self-Test

Part I

Directions: Circle the correct answer(s).

1. Which of the following is a neuroeffector transmitter?

   a serotonin *b* acetylcholine
   c norepinephrine *d* dopamine

2. A general depolarization of the membrane when excitatory synaptic activity predominates is known as

   a temporal summation. *b* facilitation.
   c IPSP. *d* convergence.

3. Synaptic delay is primarily a result of the

   a width of the synaptic cleft.
   b permeability changes in the postsynaptic membrane.
   c release mechanism which frees the transmitter.
   d time necessary for transmitter diffusion.

Part II

Directions: Circle T for true and F for false.

T F 1. An EPSP results from an increase in the membrane permeability to positively charged ions.

T F 2. Serotonin is a neuroeffector transmitter.

T F 3. An inhibitory synapse (IPSP) leads to a slight depolarization of the postsynaptic membrane.

T F 4. Synaptic events last the same length of time as an action potential.

T F 5. The flexion reflex is classed as polysynaptic because it contains interneurons between afferent and efferent nerves.

Part III

Directions: Complete the following items in the space provided.

1. Membrane-enclosed structures which contain the transmitter are termed

   ______________________.
2. Summation due to EPSPs at different places on the postsynaptic neuron is called

   ______________________.
3. Chemicals released from efferent neurons to alter the activity of glands or muscle cells are

   known as ______________________.
4. A synapse can conduct only in one direction because the

   ______________________ is on one side and the

   ______________________ are on the other.
5. A slight depolarization of the cell membrane which leads to a decrease in the amplitude of an action potential before it reaches the synapse is termed

   ______________________.

Module VI: Divisions of the Nervous System

Objectives

Upon completion of this module, the student will be able to:

1. Describe the anatomy and function of neurons in the afferent division of the peripheral nervous system.

2. Compare the neurons of the autonomic nervous system with those of the somatic nervous system.
3. Compare the sympathetic with the parasympathetic division of the autonomic nervous system.
4. Define *acetylcholine, thoracolumbar division, craniosacral division, cholinergic, norepinephrine, adrenergic, parasympatho-* and *sympathomimetic, parasympatho-* and *sympatholytic,* and *adrenal medulla.*
5. Define and give an example of *dual innervation,* and compare dual innervation with reciprocal innervation.
6. Define and locate on a diagram of the brain or spinal cord the gray matter, white matter, dorsal and ventral roots, brain stem, reticular formation, cerebellum, cerebrum, cerebral cortex, subcortical nuclei, thalamus, and hypothalamus.
7. Define *blood-brain barrier phenomena, cerebral ventricles,* and *cerebrospinal fluid.*

Reading Assignment

Chap. 6, pp. 162–171.

Supplementary Materials

The table on autonomic innervations (below) lists autonomic effects on various organs.

Structure	Sympathetic Response	Parasympathetic Response	Notes
Eyes	Dilate pupils	Constrict pupils	
Heart	Increase heart rate	Decrease heart rate	+ or − chronotropic effect
	Increase contractility	Decrease contractility	+ or − inotropic effect
Stomach and intestines	Decrease motility, secretion	Increase motility, secretion	
Adrenal medulla	Secretion	None	Innervated by preganglionic fibers (therefore cholinergic)*
Bladder	Relax bladder, constrict sphinctor	Constrict bladder, relax sphinctor	
Thermoregulatory sweat glands	Secretion	None	Cholinergic
Skin blood vessels	Vasoconstriction	None	
Skeletal-muscle blood vessels	Vasodilation	None	

* *Cholinergic:* fibers that cause effects similar to those induced by acetylcholine.

Exercises

Part I

Directions: Complete the following outline of the major division of the nervous system. Then answer the following questions in the spaces provided. (*163*)

I. Central Nervous System (CNS)
II.
  A. Afferent
  B.
    1.
    2.
      a
      b sympathetic

1. Which of the above groups conveys information from receptors to the CNS?

   ________________ Where are its cell bodies located? ________

   ____

2. Which group leaves the CNS to innervate skeletal muscle? ____________

   ____

   How many neurons are in this pathway? ________________

3. Which of the autonomic fibers are also known as the thoracolumbar division? ________

   ____

   Where do their cell bodies lie in relation to the spinal cord?

   This system functions in what type of situation?

   Give an example.

Part II

In the spaces provided, label the corresponding structures in Fig. W-12. (*169*)

A ________________ B ________________

C ________________ D ________________

E ________________

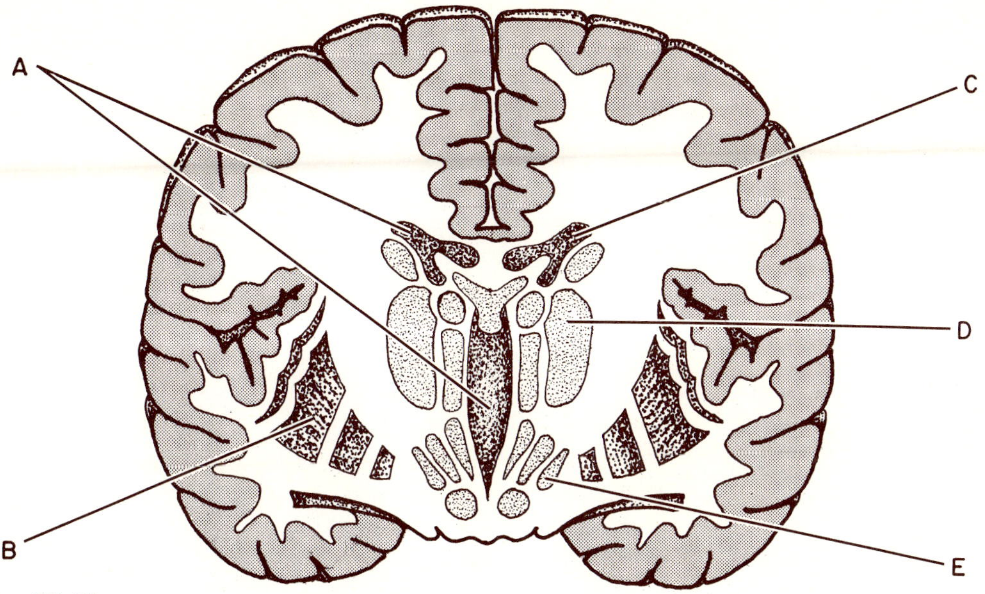

Fig. W-12

Self-Test

Part I

Directions: Circle T for true and F for false.

T F 1. Organs which are innervated by both the sympathetic and parasympathetic systems are said to receive dual innervation.

T F 2. Somatic efferent neurons synapse just outside the spinal cord prior to reaching the effector organs.

T F 3. The transmitter released from the sympathetic fibers at the effector organ is acetylcholine.

T F 4. Afferent information enters the spinal cord through the dorsal roots.

T F 5. Parasympathetic effects on the heart are to decrease heart rate and increase contractility.

Part II

Directions: Complete the following items in the space provided.

1. Another name for the parasympathetic system is the

   ______________________ division.

2. Most ascending and descending tracts are located in the

   ______________________ of the spinal cord.

3. Drugs which block the action of the parasympathetic fibers are termed

   ______________________.

4. Inhibition of the antagonist of an active muscle is known as

    ____________________________________.

5. The reticular formation is located in the ____________________________________.

Part III

Directions: Circle the correct answer(s).

1. Which of the following responses is (are) parasympathetic?

    a dilation of the pupils
    b increased stomach motility
    c vasoconstriction in the skin
    d relaxation of the urinary bladder

2. Which of the following responses is (are) sympathetic?

    a secretion by the adrenal medulla
    b decreased contractility of the heart
    c relaxation of the bladder sphincter
    d vasodilation to skeletal muscle

3. An important integrating center for most sensory input on its way to the cortex is the

    a basal ganglia. *b* cerebellum.
    c thalamus. *d* hypothalamus.

4. Which of the following has its chief role in the unconscious coordination of muscle movement?

    a reticular formation *b* cerebellum
    c thalamus *d* cerebrum

Module I:
Basics of Hormonal Control

Module II:
Pituitary Gland and Adrenal Medulla

HORMONAL CONTROL MECHANISMS

CHAPTER 7

Module I: Basics of Hormonal Control

Objectives

Upon completion of this module, the student will be able to:

1. Distinguish between endocrine and exocrine glands.
2. Define *hormone, parahormone, target-hormone cell.*
3. State the significance of target-hormone specificity.
4. List the general factors that determine the blood concentrations of hormones, such as rate of secretion and rates of inactivation and excretion.
5. List the two categories of basic cell processes commonly altered by hormones.
6. Describe the differences between direct and indirect effects of hormones.
7 Define *cyclic AMP* and describe its role in the mechanism of action of many hormones.
8. Compare the mechanism of action of steroid hormones with hormones that utilize cyclic AMP.
9. Describe the phenomenon of permissiveness and of the pharmacological effects of hormones.

Reading Assignment

Chap. 7, pp. 172–179.

Exercises

Part I

Directions: Circle T for true and F for false.

T F 1. The endocrine glands secrete hormones, whereas the exocrine glands secrete parahormones. *(172)*

T F 2. Like the nervous system, in which there is tonic activity which can be either increased or decreased, hormones are generally secreted at some rate above zero, even when not stimulated. *(173)*

T F 3. The plasma concentration of a hormone is entirely dependent upon the rate of hormone secretion. *(173)*

T F 4. The two general categories of processes commonly altered by hormones are the alteration of the activity of some essential enzyme, and the alteration of membrane transport of some substance. *(175–176)*

T F 5. Activated adenyl cyclase acts as a catalyst to transform ATP to cyclic ATP. *(177)*

T F 6. Both the cyclic AMP mechanism of hormone action and the steroid mechanism of hormone action rely on fixed receptor sites on the outer cell membrane of the target-organ cells. *(178)*

Part II

Directions: Complete the following items in the space provided.

1. The general factors which determine the blood concentrations of hormones are

   __________________________, __________________________,

   and __________________________. (*173*)
2. Sometimes known as "second messenger," this molecule transformed from ATP by the action of activated adenyl cyclase is __________________________. (*177*)
3. Administration of very large quantities of a hormone may have results which are never seen in a normal person; these are called __________________________ effects. (*178–179*)
4. Hormones which must be present (usually in small quantities) to enable other hormones to exert their full effect exhibit the phenomenon known as

   __________________________. (*178*)

Self-Test

Part I

Directions: Circle T for true and F for false.

T F 1. Secretions from both endocrine and exocrine glands act by altering enzyme activity or membrane transport.

T F 2. In the cyclic AMP mechanism of hormone action, the endocrine glands' hormonal secretion is the first messenger.

T F 3. The first messenger in the cyclic AMP mechanism of hormone action enters the cell and activates adenyl cyclase.

T F 4. Adenyl cyclase catalyzes the conversion of ATP to cyclic 3′, 5′-AMP.

T F 5. Cyclic 3′, 5′-AMP acts as the second messenger, causing an alteration in cell function associated with the particular hormone (first messenger).

T F 6. Pharmacological effects of hormones are only produced experimentally.

Part II

Directions: Circle the correct answer(s).

1. In a second-messenger system, which of the following are *not* correct.
   a The activating hormone (first messenger) interacts with a receptor site on the cell membrane.
   b The activating hormone activates adenyl cyclase.
   c Activated adenyl cyclase catalyzes the transformation of ATP to cyclic AMP.
   d The cyclic AMP acts inside the cell to alter the cell function as characteristic for the specific hormone.
2. Which of the following are true for the mechanism of action of a steroid hormone?
   a passes through the cell membrane into the cell cytoplasm
   b interacts with a receptor site on the cell membrane to activate adenyl cyclase

c binds to a hormone-specific soluble cytoplasmic protein known as the receptor
d results in transformation of ATP to cyclic AMP
e hormone-protein complex moves into the cell nucleus and triggers RNA synthesis
f is known as the mobile receptor system

Module II: Pituitary Gland and Adrenal Medulla

Objectives

Upon completion of this module, the student will be able to:

1. List each of the major endocrine glands and the hormones they produce. The endocrine glands to be considered are the anterior and posterior pituitary, thyroid, parathyroid, adrenal gland, pancreas, gonads, and kidneys.
2. Identify the two lobes of the pituitary and their relationship (physical connection) to the hypothalamus.
3. Identify the characteristics of the hypothalamopituitary system by identifying the mechanism providing for communication between the hypothalamus and the anterior pituitary.
4. Identify the function served by a "releasing factor."
5. List the five hypothalamic releasing factors and the one inhibiting factor.
6. Describe the neural and hormonal controls of releasing-factor secretion by completing a diagram similar to the one in Fig. 7-12, p. 184.
7. Predict the effects of hypothalamic lesions, pituitary destruction, pituitary transplantation to a distant site in the body, and changes in hormone excretion (including inactivation) on the rates of secretion of releasing factors, pituitary hormones, and target gland hormones.
8. Identify the mechanism of the posterior pituitary hypothalamic system that controls secretion of oxytocin and ADH by stating the origin of the posterior pituitary, the location of oxytocin and ADH synthesis, those mechanisms by which ADH and oxytocin move from the hypothalamus to the posterior pituitary, and the mechanism controlling the release of ADH and oxytocin into the blood.
9. Identify the mechanism controlling epinephrine secretion by the adrenal medulla.

Reading Assignment

Chap. 7, pp. 179–188.

Exercises

Directions: Answer the following questions concerning a person whose anterior pituitary has been removed.

1. Will the person be fertile? ______________________ Why or why not?

2. What will be the effect on the

   a thyroid gland ______________________________

   ____

   b adrenal cortex ______________________________

   ____

   c testes ______________________________

   ____

3. Will releasing factors continue to be produced? (*180–185*)

   ____

Self-Test

Part I

Directions: Circle the correct answer(s).

1. Which of the following hormones are produced by the anterior pituitary?

   a insulin *b* growth hormone (GH)
   c testosterone *d* ACTH

2. The pancreas produces which of the following hormones?

   a insulin *b* glucagon
   c ACTH *d* TSH-releasing factor

3. The anterior pituitary

   a is an outgrowth of the hypothalamus.
   b is composed of neural tissue.
   c produces TSH and ACTH.
   d is composed of glandular tissue.

4. Following surgical removal of the hypothalamic area responsible for the secretion of the so-called releasing factors, which of the following would occur?

   a blood levels of prolactin decrease
   b blood levels of thyroxin increase
   c size of testes decrease
   d plasma growth-hormone levels decrease

Part II

Directions: Complete the following items in the space provided.

1. What are the two lobes of the pituitary called?

   a ______________________ *b* ______________________

2. Name the system that provides for communication between the hypothalamus and the anterior pituitary. ______________________

3. Describe the method of communication used by the system in question 2 above.

4. What function does a releasing factor serve? ______________________

____

____

5. List the five releasing factors and one inhibiting factor.

   a ______________________

   b ______________________

   c ______________________

   d ______________________

   e ______________________

   f ______________________

6. Trace the neural pathway controlling secretion of ACTH. Your answer may be verbal or diagrammatic or both. (See Fig. W-13 in the Answer Key.)

Part III

Directions: Complete the accompanying chart to show the effects certain events have on the rates of secretion of releasing factors, pituitary hormones, and target hormones.

	Effects on Rates of Secretion of		
Events	Releasing Factors	Pituitary Hormones	Target Gland Hormones
1. Hypothalamic lesions			
2. Pituitary destruction			
3. Pituitary transplantation to a distant site in the body			
4. Increase in pituitary hormone secretion			
5. Decrease in pituitary hormone secretion			

Part IV

Directions: Circle T for true and F for false.

T F 1. The posterior pituitary is an outgrowth of the anterior pituitary.
T F 2. Oxytocin and ADH are synthesized within the posterior pituitary.
T F 3. Epinephrine is secreted by the adrenal medulla.
T F 4. Epinephrine secretion is dependent upon stimulation of sympathetic nerves.

CHAPTER 8 MUSCLE

Module I:
Muscle Structure

Module II:
Muscle Contraction

Module III:
Metabolism of Muscle

Module I: Muscle Structure

Objectives

Upon completion of this module, the student will be able to:

1. Define the term *striated muscle.*
2. Diagram a skeletal muscle fiber and identify the functional elements, including the sarcomere, thin myofilament comprised of actin, thick myofilament comprised of myosin, Z line, H zone, A band, I band, and cross bridges.
3. Describe the mechanical changes in muscle structure during contraction according to the Huxley sliding filament model.
4. Describe the changes in the A, I, and H bands during contraction and relate these to the Huxley sliding filament model.
5. Identify the role of ATP in the movement of myofibrils, both in contraction and relaxation.

Reading Assignment

Chap. 8, pp. 189–195.

Exercises

Part I

Directions: Using Fig. W-14, label the following structures:

a thin filament | *b* thick filament | *c* sarcomere
d H zone | *e* I band | *f* A band
g Z line | *h* cross bridges

Identify the function of each of the above during contraction and relaxation. (See Fig. 8-2, p. 192, for help.)

Part II

Directions: Draw a cross section of a myofibril. Use large dots to represent thick filaments, and small dots to represent thin filaments. Indicate the location of the cross bridges. See Fig. 8-3, p. 193, to check your answer.

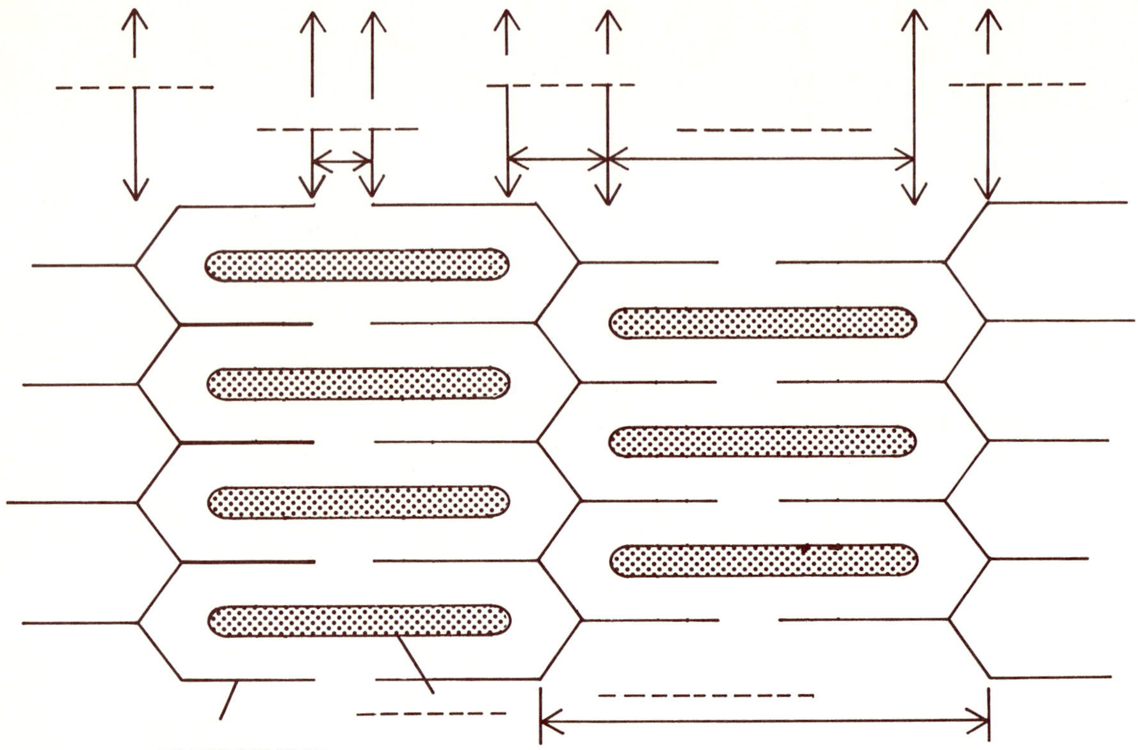

Fig. W-14 Fibrillar organization.

Self-Test

Part I

Directions: Circle T for true and F for false.

T F 1. Blood vessels and nerve fibers surround individual skeletal muscle fibers.
T F 2. In certain muscles, the tendons provide part of the contractile force.
T F 3. The striated appearance of skeletal muscles is caused by the arrangement of myofibrils.

Part II

Directions: Complete the following items in the space provided.

1. What type of muscle surrounds the stomach, bladder, and intestines?

   ____

2. How many thin filaments are arranged around each thick filament in cross-sectional micrograph? ______________________________

3. What proteins are present in the thick filament ______________________________, and the thin filament ______________________________?

Part III

Directions: Circle the correct answer(s).

1. Which structures of a contracting muscle fiber decrease in size?

   a sarcomere *b* H zone *c* I band
   d A band *e* Z line *f* cross bridges

2. Which element below is indicated by the A band?

   a sarcomere *b* thick filament
   c thin filament *d* Z line

Part IV

Directions: Identify each of the following three equations as representative of the interaction during actin binding, bridge contraction, or bridge relaxation.

1. ______________________ $A \cdot M \cdot ATP \longrightarrow A \cdot M + ADP + Pi$

2. ______________________ $A + M \cdot ATP \longrightarrow A \cdot M \cdot ATP$

3. ______________________ $A \cdot M + ATP \longrightarrow A + M \cdot ATP$

Module II: **Muscular Contraction**

Objectives

Upon completion of this module, the student will be able to:

1. Identify the elements responsible for excitation-contraction coupling, including sarcolemma, sarcoplasmic reticulum, lateral sacs, transverse tubules, and troponin and tropomyosin.
2. Describe the events that occur at an active neuromuscular junction, including a discussion of the motor end plate, acetylcholine, end-plate potential, acetylcholine-esterase, and muscle-action potential.
3. Identify the roles of the elements listed in objective 1 above during excitation, contraction, relaxation, making particular note of Ca^{2+} movement. (See Fig. 8-14, p. 201.)
4. Identify a muscular contraction as isotonic or isometric.
5. Identify the structures and functions of the series elastic component and the causes of summation.
6. Identify the characteristics of isotonic and isometric twitches in regard to latency, contraction time, relaxation time, and duration. (See Fig. 8-18, p. 205.)
7. Identify the relationships of tension developed or distance shortened in summation and tetanus during an isotonic and isometric contraction.
8. Define the terms *motor unit, recruitment of motor unit, length tension relationship,* and *lever action.*
9. Graph the relation between length and tension. State this relation in terms of the sliding filament model.

Reading Assignment

Chap. 8, pp. 196–212, particularly Table 8-1, p. 204.

Exercises

Part I

Directions: Fill in the missing information in the following sequence of events between a nerve action potential and muscle contraction and relaxation. (See Table 8-1, p. 204.)

1. The action potential in the motor neuron causes release at the neuromuscular junction of ______________________________ ______________________________.
2. Acetylcholine is bound to reactive sites on the ______________________________ membrane.
3. Acetylcholine causes a permeability change producing a(n) ______________________________ potential.
4. The muscle membrane is depolarized and a muscle action potential is generated over the surface of the muscle ______________________________.
5. Acetylcholine is rapidly destroyed on the end-plate membrane by ______________________________ ______________________________.
6. The muscle action potential, at the A-I junction of the sarcomeres, depolarizes______________________________ ______________________________.
7. This depolarization leads the lateral sacs of the sarcoplasmic reticulum surrounding the myofibrils to release ______________________________.
8. Ca^{2+} binds on the thin actin filament to ______________________________.
9. This binding releases the inhibition that prevents actin from binding to myosin ______________________________.
10. $A + M \cdot ATP \longrightarrow$ ______________________________.
11. $A \cdot M \cdot ATP \longrightarrow A \cdot M \cdot ADP + P$; and causes movement of the ______________________________.
12. The actin-myosin bond is broken, allowing the cross bridge to relax, when ATP exchanges with ______________________________.
13. Inhibition of the cross-bridge contraction and relaxation cycles occurs with a drop in the concentration of ______________________________.
14. The Ca^{2+} level drops as ATP is split and Ca^{2+} returns to the ______________________________.

Part II

1. The length at which the muscle develops the maximum tension is l_0. What are the two factors that lead to decreased tension at shorter lengths? (209)

   a ______________________________

   b ______________________________

2. Passively stretching a muscle changes the amount of overlap between the thick and thin filaments in the myofibrils. How would the thick and thin filaments look in the following situations?

   a at l_0 ______________________________

   b at 175 percent of l_0 ________________________ (209)

3. Classical observations and experiments proved the relationship between muscle length and the tension the muscle can develop at that length. Draw a graph to show the following pattern.

   a When the muscle is set at a length equal to

   60 percent of l_0 it develops no tension.
   78 percent of l_0 it develops 78 percent tension.
   94 percent of l_0 it develops 100 percent tension.
   110 percent of l_0 it develops 100 percent tension.
   175 percent of l_0 it develops no tension.

   b Shade the band that represents the range of muscle length changes that can occur in the body while the muscles are still attached to bones. (209)

Part III

Directions: Label the indicated structures or events on Fig. W-15. (See Fig. 8-16, p. 203.)

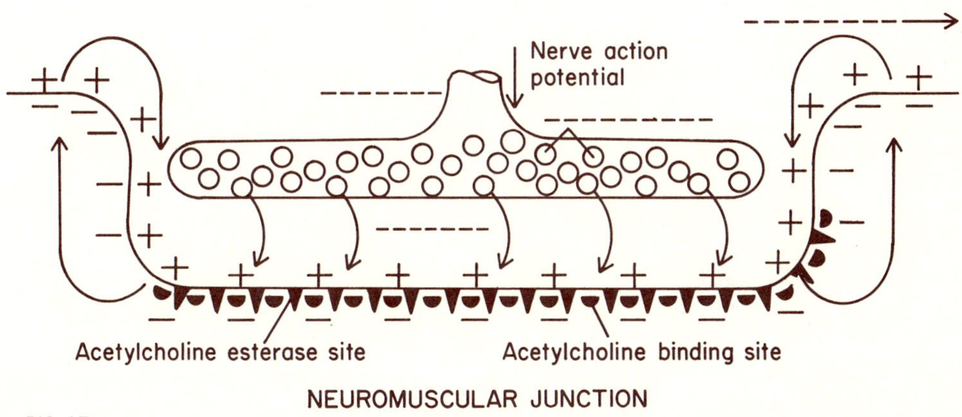

Fig. W-15

Self-Test

Part I

Directions: Circle T for true and F for false.

T F 1. Calcium ions are released from the lateral sacs when the t tubules are depolarized.

T F 2. The resting length of a muscle determines the amount of isometric tension it can develop.

T F 3. Calcium ions are returned to the lateral sacs by active transport.

T F 4. At l_0, which represents the length at which the muscle develops maximum tension, the thick and thin filaments are so far apart that there is no overlap between the two.

T F 5. A motor unit consists of the motor neuron and all the muscle fibers innervated by it.

T F 6. The motor neuron contains an esterase which inactivates acetylcholine following depolarization of the motor end plate.

T F 7. In the body, where muscles are attached to bones, the relaxed length of the muscle is at the minimal length for force generation.

Part II

Directions: Complete the following items in the space provided.

1. The action potential which initiates excitation-contraction coupling is located in the muscle ____________________.
2. The junctions between nerve fiber and skeletal muscle are known as ____________________.
3. The chemical transmitter agent released at a neuromuscular junction to initiate membrane depolarization of skeletal muscle fiber is ____________________.
4. The cell bodies of the motor neurons are located in the ____________________ and ____________________.
5. If a muscle is not allowed to relax completely between successive contractions, it is undergoing ____________________.
6. The combination of the motor neuron and the muscle fibers it innervates is known as a ____________________.

Part III

Directions: Circle the correct answer(s).

1. The transverse tubules (or t tubules) are an invagination of the

   a sarcoplasmic reticulum. *b* muscle membrane.
   c endoplasmic reticulum.

2. Tropomyosin and troponin affect myosin ATPase activity by

   a blocking the binding of calcium to myosin.
   b blocking the binding of actin to myosin.
   c inhibiting the uptake of calcium by the sarcoplasmic reticulum.

3. Tropomyosin and troponin can be found in the

   a thick filaments. *b* thin filaments.
   c H band. *d* transverse tubule.

4. A twitch does *not* include

   a a mechanical response.
   b an electrical response.
   c anything other than isometric contractions.
   d a response to a single, induced stimulus.

5. The elastic component of the three-component model plays an important role in

   a fatigue. *b* aging. *c* summation.

Part IV

Directions: Each of the graphs in Fig. W-16 is characteristic of an isotonic or isometric twitch. Label each graph and circle the correct parameter for each.

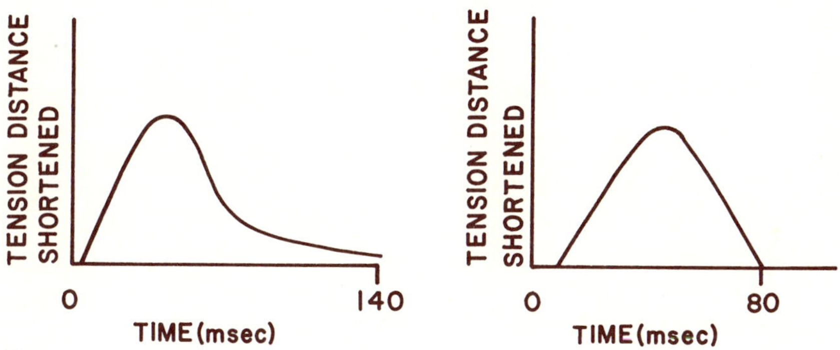

Fig. W-16

Module III: Metabolism of Muscle

Objectives

Upon completion of this module, the student will be able to:

1. Identify three major functions of ATP in cross-bridge movement (see Fig. 8-10, p. 197).
2. Identify three sources of ATP in active muscle (see Fig. 8-31, p. 215).
3. Identify the three major functions of ATP in contraction and relaxation of muscle.
4. Describe the factors that limit the replacement of ATP by oxidative phosphorylation.
5. Define *denervation atrophy, disuse atrophy,* and *hypertrophy.*
6. List the three classes of skeletal muscle on the basis of the rate of utilization of ATP.
7. Define *myoglobin* and state its functional significance.
8. Describe the relationships between heat, work, and efficiency in muscle.
9. Compare the changes produced in muscle by high-tension, low-frequency exercise, with those produced by low-tension, high-frequency exercise.
10. Identify the differences and similarities in skeletal, cardiac, and smooth muscle according to the supplementary material.
11. Differentiate between single-unit and multiunit smooth muscle, and include a discussion of the significance of the gap junction.
12. Define and describe the pacemaker potential and give examples of its occurrence.

Reading Assignment

Chap. 8, pp. 212–225.

Supplementary Materials

See Table I, which shows the three types of muscle.

Exercises

1. Complete Table II by giving the name of the right type of muscle, according to the different properties (see the supplemental materials for help).
2. Complete Table III (p.70) to show some of the characteristics of the three types of skeletal muscle fibers. *(219)*
3. Suppose you are doing calisthenics to build up your body. Your muscles really get tired after each session. You know very intense exercise causes breakdown of ATP. Three factors begin to limit the replacement of ATP by oxidative phosphorylation. What are these three factors? *(214)*

   a ____________________

   b ____________________

   c ____________________

Table I

Properties	Skeletal	Cardiac	Smooth
Sarcomere organization	Rigid	Rigid	Loose
Dependence on nerve	Absolute	Regulatory	Regulatory and absolute
Myogenic activity	None	Some	Most
Dependence on muscle-action potential to contract	Absolute	Absolute	Variable
Cell-to-cell propagation (nexuses)	Absent	Present	Most, but variable
Humoral influence	Minimal	Great	Great
Refractory period	Very short	Long	Variable
Speed of contraction	Fast	Intermediate	Slow
Autorhythmicity	None	All	Some
Neuromuscular junctions	Present	Specialized	Variable, but most
Tetanic contraction	Yes	No	No, modified
Resting membrane potential	Stable	Depolarizing (pacemaker potential)	Stable and variable

Table II

Properties	Type of Muscle
Rigid sarcomere organization Minimal humoral influence Fast contraction speed No nexuses	
No tetanic contraction Specialized neuromuscular junctions Long refractory period Absolute dependence on action potential	
Absolute dependence on nerve No myogenic activity No autorhythmicity Stable resting membrane potential	
Great humoral influence Variable refractory period Stable and variable resting membrane potential Slow contraction speed	
Loose sarcomere organization Regulatory and absolute dependence on nerve No or modified tetanic contraction Some autorhythmicity	

Table III

	High-oxidative Fast-twitch	Low-oxidative Fast-twitch	High-oxidative Slow-twitch
Rate of fatigue		Fast	
Glycolytic enzyme activity		High	
Fiber diameter		Large	
Myoglobin content		Low	
Capillaries		Few	

Self-Test

Part I

Directions: Complete the following items in the space provided.

1. The increase in the size of the individual muscle fibers caused by increased amounts of neural activity is called ____________________.
2. The capacity of a muscle for activity can be altered in two ways. List them.
   a ____________________
   b ____________________
3. The decrease in muscle mass following denervation is known as what type of atrophy?
   ____
4. A muscle can atrophy with its nerve supply intact if it is not used for a long time, and this is known as what type of atrophy? ____________________
5. In a single-unit smooth muscle, the spontaneous depolarization of the membrane which occurs at regular intervals is known as a ____________________
6. The three sources of ATP in active muscle are
   a ____________________
   b ____________________
   c ____________________

Part II

Directions: Circle T for true and F for false.

T F 1. In multiunit smooth muscles, the contractile activity can be initiated by electrical activity in the nerve fibers to the muscle.

T F 2. Cardiac muscle is a striated muscle having myofibrils with thick and thin myofilaments.

T F 3. When contraction is initiated, the myosin ATPase breaks down ATP at a very low rate.

T F 4. Creatine phosphate provides the most rapid means of forming ATP in the muscle cell.

Part III

Directions: Circle the correct answer(s).

1. Which of the following could be found in cardiac muscle?

   a striations
   b myofibrils with thick and thin myofilaments
   c poorly developed sarcoplasmic reticulum
   d gap junctions

2. Anaerobic glycolysis requires

   a large quantities of glucose.
   b small quantities of glucose.
   c no glucose.

3. High-oxidative fibers have which of the following characteristics?

   a few mitochondria in the fiber
   b myoglobin in the fiber
   c many surrounding capillaries
   d high rate of oxidative phosphorylation

4. The protein myoglobin

   a binds oxygen and increases the rate of oxygen diffusion into the muscle cell.
   b is red.
   c provides a mechanism for storing oxygen within the muscle.
   d is found in white cells of the blood.

CHAPTER 9 CIRCULATION

Module I:
General Functions and Design of the Circulatory System

Module II:
The Function of the Heart as a Pump

Module III:
Factors in Cardiac Output

Module IV:
The Vascular System, Part I

Module V:
The Vascular System, Part II

Module VI:
Integration of Cardiovascular Function

Module VII:
Cardiovascular Patterns in Health and Disease

Module I: General Functions and Design of the Circulatory System

Objectives

Upon completion of this module, the student will be able to:

1. Identify the following elements transported by the blood: oxygen, carbon dioxide, nutrients, wastes, hormones, electrolytes, proteins, vitamins, and heat.
2. Define and explain the relationships between the circulatory system and diffusion, net transport, internal environment, ultrafiltration, and arborization (branching).
3. Make a line drawing of the heart with arrows indicating the path of blood flow. The drawing will include the superior and inferior venae cavae, left and right atria, left and right ventricles, pulmonary veins and artery, and aorta.
4. Define and give average values for hematocrit, plasma volume, and total blood volume.

Reading Assignment

Chap. 9, pp. 228–233. Pay particular attention to Fig. 9-2 and Fig. 9-3. Also see pp. 254–260 on capillaries and diffusion.

Supplementary Materials

See Fig. W-17.

Exercises

Directions: In Fig. W-18, label the four chambers of the heart. (Indicate *left* or *right*.) Label all veins and arteries shown. Trace the flow of blood through the heart. (See Figs. 9-3, 9-4, and 9-5; pp. 232–233.)

Self-Test

Part I

Directions: Complete the following items in the space provided.

1. Four important substances transported by the blood are

   a ______________________ *b* ______________________

   c ______________________ *d* ______________________

2. Write the name of the appropriate body part in each empty rectangle of Fig. W-19. (Answer Key Fig. W-20 shows correct labeling.)

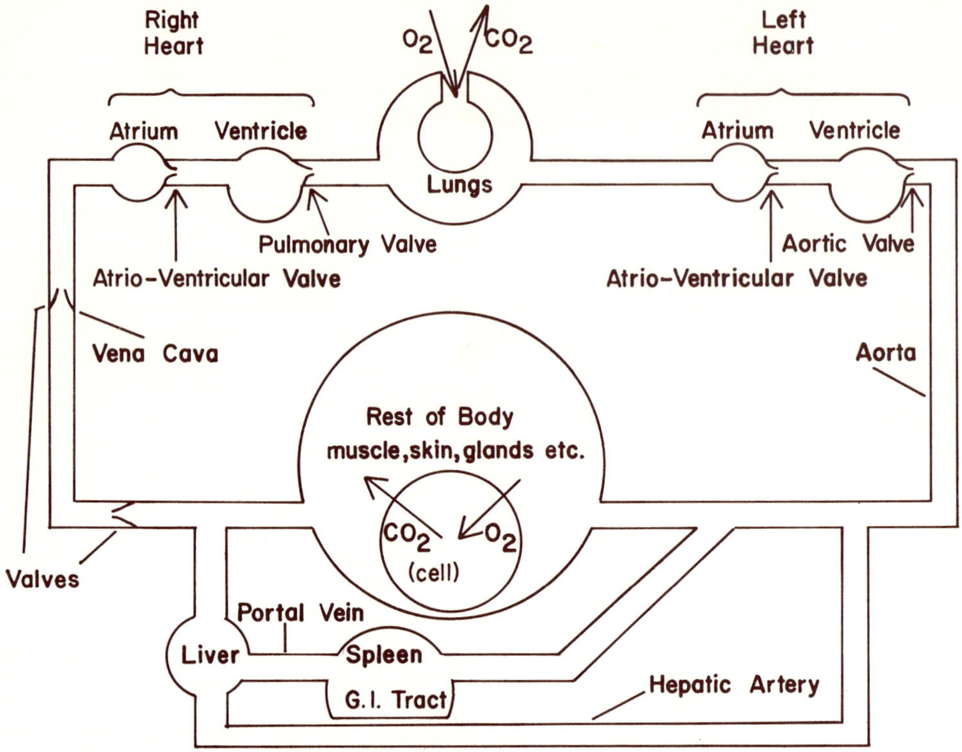

Fig. W-17 Schematic diagram of the flow of blood.

3. How many valves are there in the heart? ______________________________
4. Make a line drawing of the heart. Include and label the

   a left and right atria.
   b left and right ventricles.
   c aorta.
   d pulmonary veins and artery.
   e superior and inferior venae cavae.

Part II

Directions: Circle T for true and F for false.

T F 1. The percentage of total blood volume which is plasma is known as the hematocrit.

T F 2. The total blood volume of a person weighing 70 kg is approximately 3 liters.

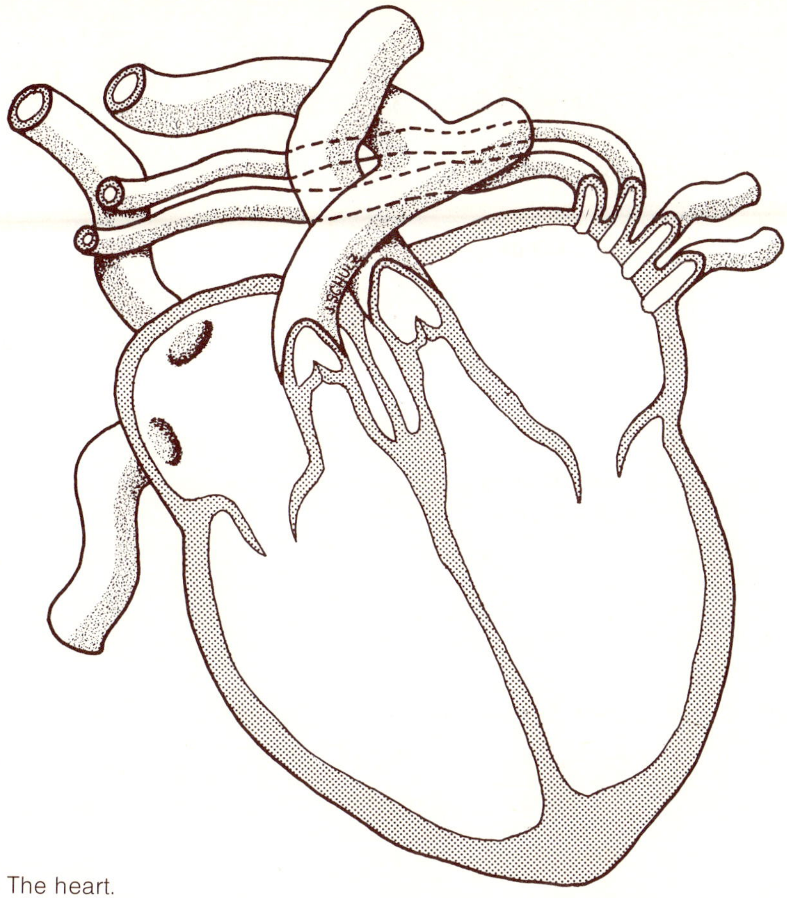

Fig. W-18 The heart.

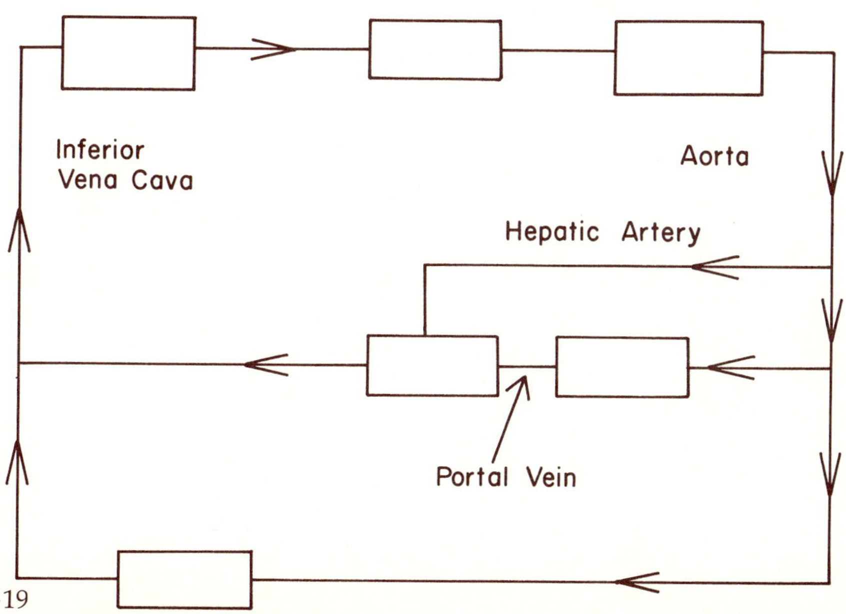

Fig. W-19

Module II: The Function of the Heart as a Pump

Objectives

After completing this module, the student will be able to:

1. List in sequence the structures activated by the "wave of excitation" in a normal heartbeat. These will include the sinoatrial (SA) node, right and left atrial muscles, atrioventricular (AV) node, Purkinje system and bundle of His, and right and left ventricular muscles.
2. Label, on a line drawing of the heart, and state the function of the superior vena cava, SA node, AV node, right bundle branches, and left bundle branches.
3. Specify the role of the refractory period in a normal and abnormal (such as asynchrony, fibrillation, increased excitability) heartbeat.
4. Identify a normal ECG and relate it to corresponding heart action, including the P wave, QRS complex, and T wave.
5. Diagram the mechanical steps in a heartbeat, including the five steps shown at the bottom of Fig. 9-15, p. 239, and describing blood flow at each phase, valve action, relative pressure in each chamber, chambers contracting. Identify each mechanical step as either diastole or systole.
6. Define *coronary blood vessels,* and state their function.

Reading Assignment

Chap. 9, pp. 233–241. Pay particular attention to Figs. 9-8, 9-10, 9-13, and 9-15.

Exercises

Directions: Label the P, Q, R, S, and T portions of the ECG in Fig. W-21. Draw a dotted line representing the ventricular contraction. (Fig. 9-13, p. 238.)

Self-Test

Part I

1. On Fig. W-22, shade the areas that are excited at the beginning phase of ventricular excitation. Label (*a*) the superior vena cava, (*b*) the sinoatrial node, (*c*) the atrioventricular node, (*d*) the right bundle branches, and (*e*) the left bundle branches.
2. On the axis in Fig. W-23, draw a normal ECG within the stage given. Label the P wave, QRS complex, and the T wave. (Fig. W-25, in the Answer Key, shows correct labeling.)

Part II

Directions: Circle T for true and F for false.

T F 1. Blood flows from the ventricles during the entire ventricular contraction.

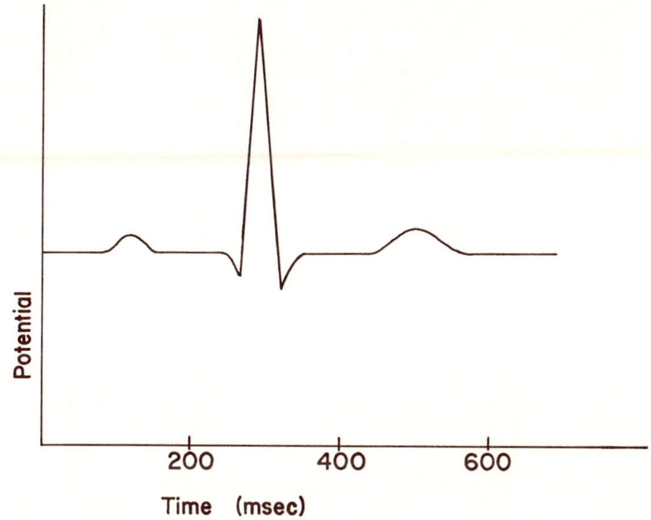

Fig. W-21 Electrocardiogram.

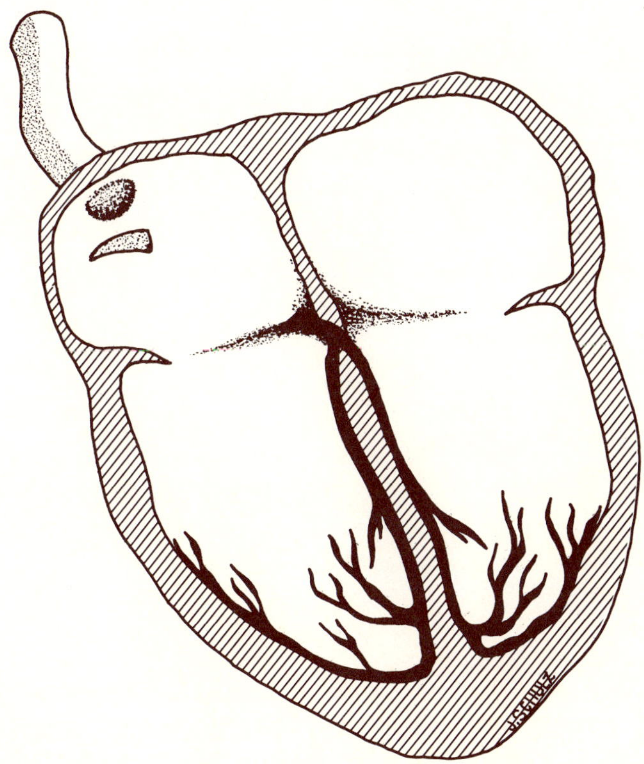

Fig. W-22

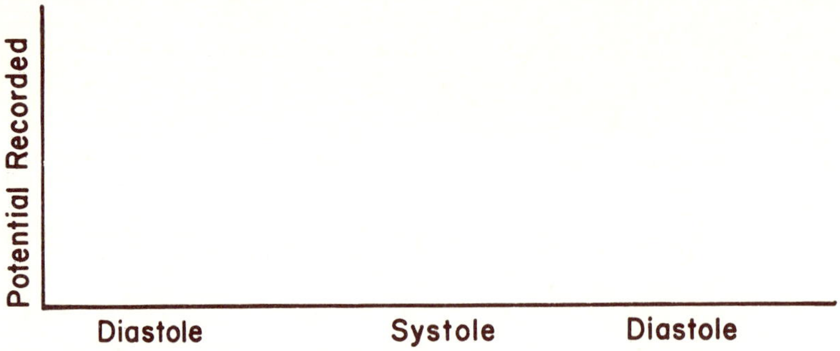

Fig. W-23

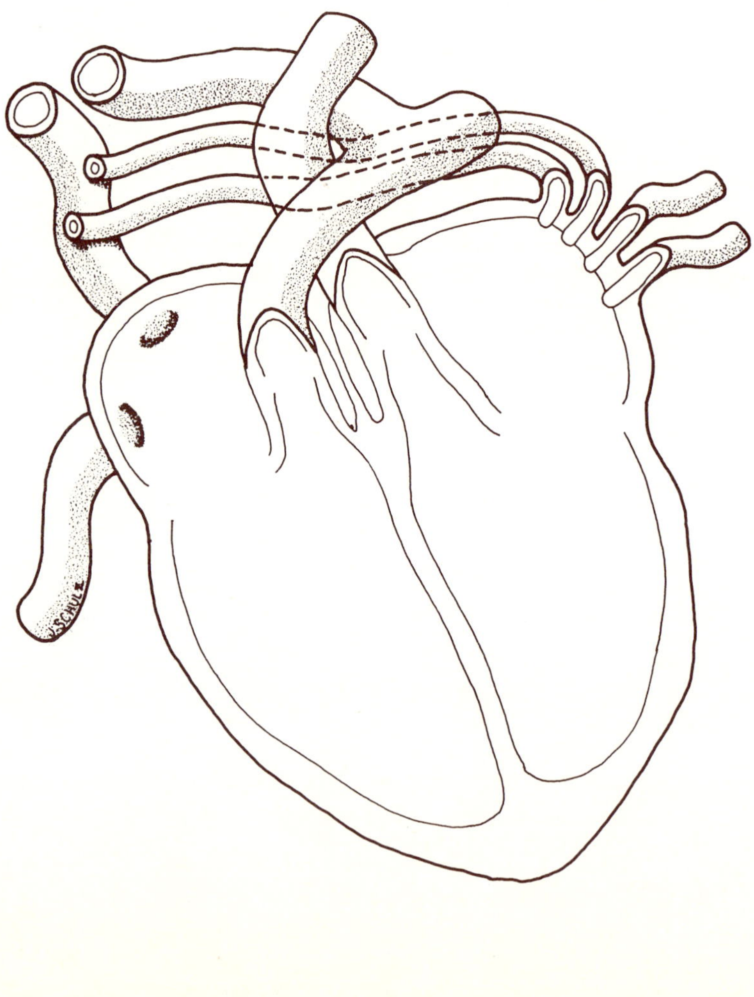

Fig. W-24

T F 2. Blood flows from the atria during the entire atrial contraction.
T F 3. The ventricles will contract only if stimulated by action potentials arising from the sinoatrial node.

Part III

Directions: On Fig. W-24:

1. Indicate (by shading) the portion of the heart muscle contracting during isovolumetric contraction at the beginning of ventricular systole.
2. Draw in valves opening into the correct areas. Indicate with arrows the movement of blood through the appropriate openings during mid-diastole. (Answer Key Fig. W-26 shows correct shading and arrows.)

Module III: Factors in Cardiac Output

Objectives

Upon completion of this module, the student will be able to:

1. Define *cardiac output* (CO), *heart rate* (HR), and *stroke volume* (SV), and identify normal values for each.
2. Calculate any of the variables in the following formula, given the other two:

$$\underset{\text{(ml/min)}}{\text{CO}} = \underset{\text{(beats/min)}}{\text{HR}} \times \underset{\text{(ml/beat)}}{\text{SV}}$$

3. State how heart rate is affected by parasympathetic nerve stimulation, sympathetic nerve stimulation, epinephrine, and norepinephrine.
4. Specify the intrinsic adaptability of the heart to cope with increased blood flow by using Starling's law of the heart. (See Supplementary Materials.)
5. Define contractility as the strength of contraction at any given initial muscle-fiber length and relate active and passive length tension curves to systolic and diastolic pressures in heart.

Reading Assignment

Chap. 9, pp. 241–245; Fig. 9-23, p. 247.

Supplementary Materials

The following are the normal values for CO, HR, and SV:

$$\underset{\text{CO}}{5600 \text{ ml/min}} = \underset{\text{HR}}{70 \text{ beats/min}} \times \underset{\text{SV}}{80 \text{ ml/beat}}$$

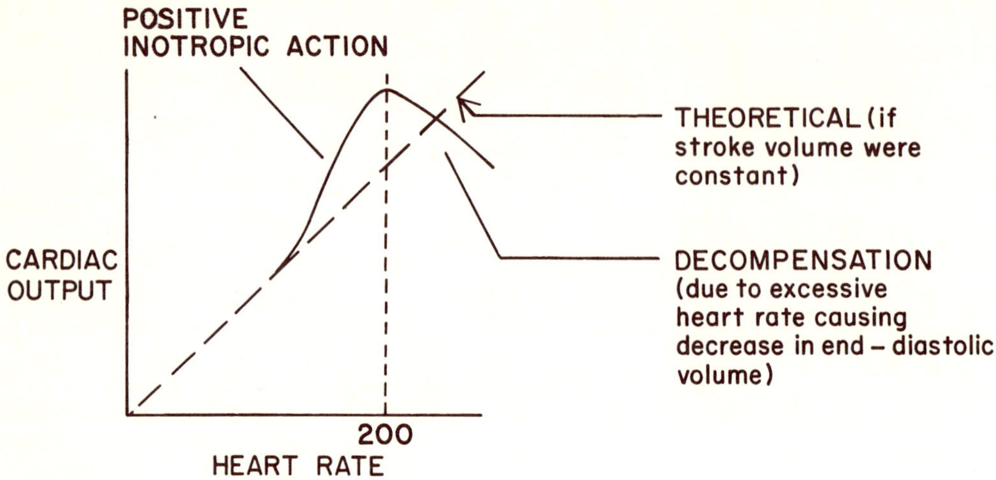

Fig. W-27

Occasionally you will encounter the terms *inotropic* (Fig. W-27) and *chronotropic* in reference to cardiac function.

Inotropic: of or pertaining to strength of contraction (either positive or negative).
Chronotropic: of or pertaining to rate of contraction (either positive or negative).

Exercises

Part I

Directions: Fill in the missing labels in Fig. W-28, which is a summary of factors that influence the cardiac output. Indicate by drawing an arrowhead on the vertical line in each box whether

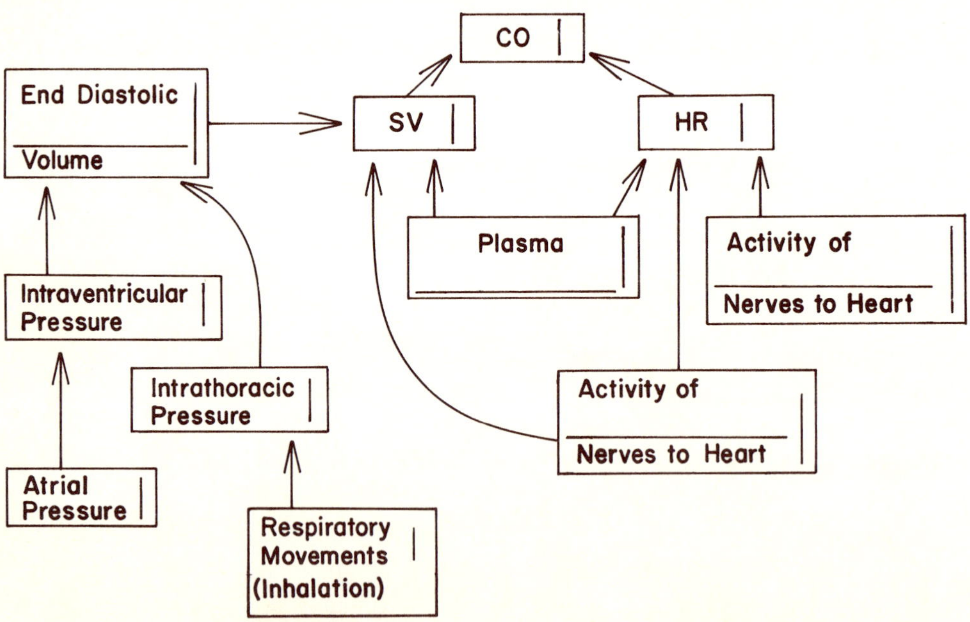

Fig. W-28 Cardiac output factors.

each factor should be increased (arrow up) or decreased (arrow down) to increase the cardiac output. (Fig. 9-23, p. 247.)

Part II

Directions: Calculate the cardiac output for a normal male patient who has a pulse of 70 beats/min and a stroke volume of 80 ml/beat. (*241*)

Self-Test

Part I

Directions: Indicate how each of the following factors directly affects cardiac output by placing an increase (↑), decrease (↓), or no change (↔) symbol in each space. Some are done for you as an example.

Factor	HR	×	SV	=	CO
1. Increased intraventricular pressure	⟷				
2. Increased parasympathetic nerve stimulation			⟷		
3. Increased sympathetic nerve stimulation					
4. Smaller respiratory movements	⟷				
5. Increased plasma epinephrine					

Part II

Directions: Circle T for true and F for false.

T F 1. Starling's law of the heart explains why the stroke volume increases to compensate for a decrease in the blood flow from the venae cavae.

T F 2. Stimulation of the parasympathetics increases the slope of the pacemaker potential which causes the cell to reach threshold more rapidly, thus increasing the heart rate.

T F 3. When inspiration decreases the intrathoracic pressure and increases the intraventricular volume, there is an increase in stroke volume.

T F 4. The difference between the end-diastolic and end-systolic volumes is 0.07 liters. This tells you that the patient's contractility is normal.

Module IV: The Vascular System, Part I

Objectives

Upon completion of this module, the student will be able to:

1. Calculate fluid flow or a variable affecting it by using the equations

$$F = kP \qquad F = \frac{\Delta P}{R} \qquad R \simeq \frac{l}{r^4}$$

where F = flow
k = flow constant
ΔP = pressure difference
R = resistance
$1/k$ = resistance
r = radius
l = length

2. Complete a graph showing the relation between cross-sectional area and the velocity of flow in the systemic circulation (as in Fig. 9-36, p. 256), and the arteries, arterioles, veins, venules, capillaries, velocity, and area.
3. Describe the concept of fluid energy and its relationship to upright posture.

Reading Assignment

Chap. 9, pp. 246–263 and 274–278. Concentrate on the principles affecting fluid flow in general and properties of the vasculature affecting blood flow.

Study Fig. 9-25, p. 248. Note the different effects doubling the length and doubling the radius have on resistance to flow.

Study Fig. 9-35, p. 255. Note that the total flow in the smaller vessels is equal to the total flow in the large vessel.

Supplementary Materials

Total fluid energy = pressure energy + gravitational potential energy + kinetic energy

$$E_{total} = P + \rho g h + \tfrac{1}{2}\rho v^2$$

where ρ = density
g = gravitational constant
v = velocity (274–278)

This equation is a more detailed statement of the concepts developed in the text. The term "kinetic energy" is generally considered small and hence is neglected in the textbook discussion.

Exercises

Part I

Directions: Answer the following items in the space provided.

1. How are the structures of the individual vessels adapted to their individual functions? *(248–254)*

2. What are the functional similarities which account for the duplication in design between lymphatics and veins? *(260–263)*

Part II

Directions: On Fig. W-29 (p. 84), identify the following parts (Fig. 9-40, p. 261).

1. arteries
2. arterioles
3. veins
4. venules
5. capillaries

Part III

Directions: Complete the graph in Fig. W-30 (p. 85) by labeling the following parts (Fig. 9-36, p. 256).

1. arteries
2. arterioles
3. veins
4. venules
5. capillaries
6. velocity
7. area

Self-Test

Part I

Directions: Complete each item in the space provided.

1. Given a vessel 10 cm long, with the initial pressure 81 mmHg and end pressure 76 mmHg, find the following if the flow is 10 ml/min:

   $R_1 =$

   If another vessel of the same diameter were 20 cm with the same ΔP, find the values for the following:

   a $k =$
   b $R_2 =$
   c $F =$

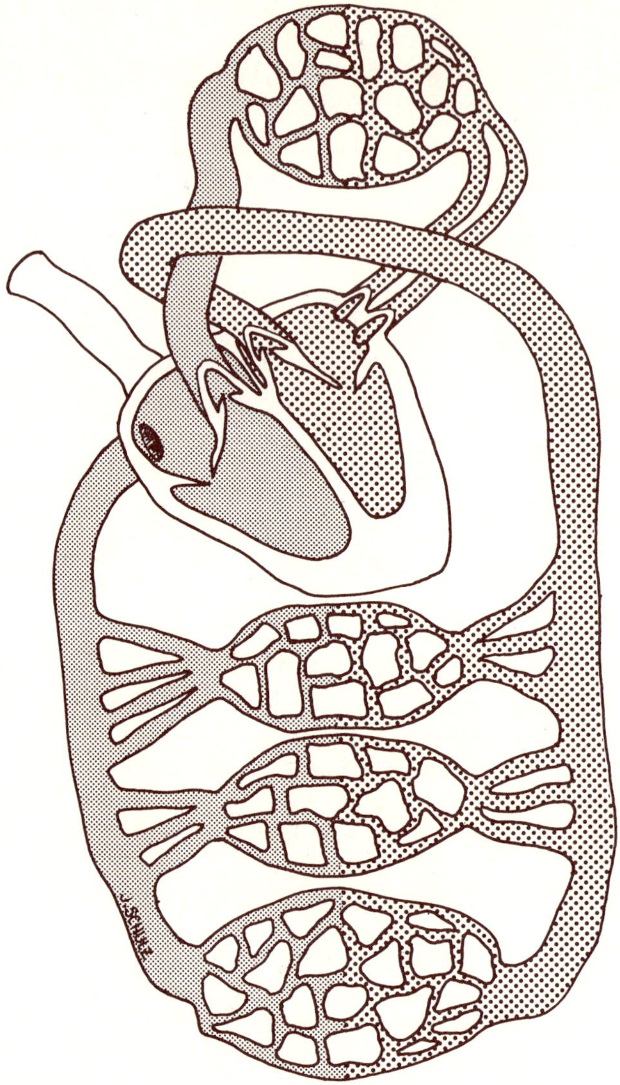

Fig. W-29 Flow of blood through the vascular system.

Part II

Directions: Circle T for true and F for false.

T F 1. The driving pressure at each artery in the systemic circulation of a recumbent human is essentially the same.

T F 2. The capillaries function by contraction of the muscle in their walls.

T F 3. The venules are muscular structures whose primary function is to restrict the flow of blood through the capillaries.

T F 4. The pulmonary circulation must have higher blood pressure because of the volume of blood being forced through it.

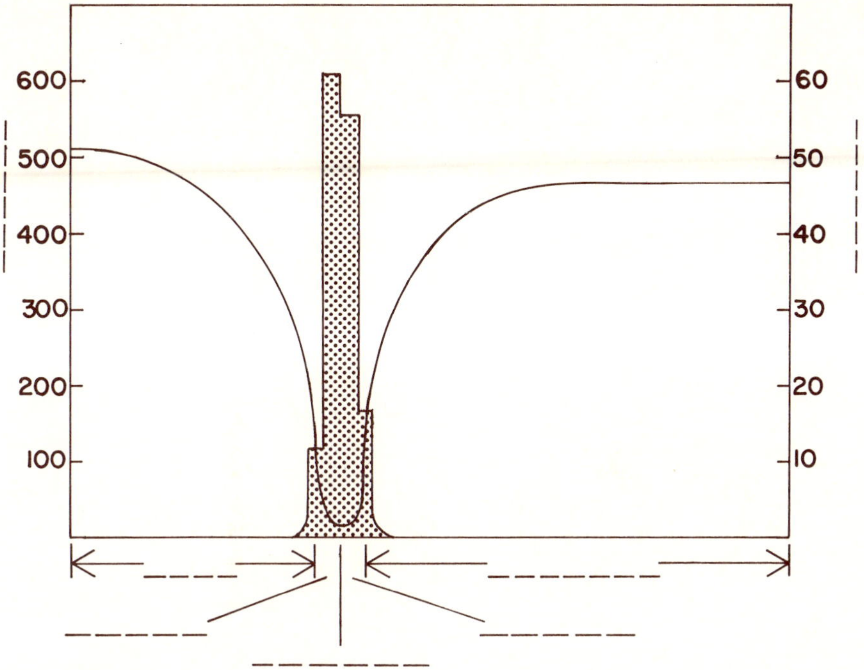

Fig. W-30 Systemic circulation.

Module V: The Vascular System, Part II

Objectives

Upon completion of this module, the student will be able to:

1. List the major effects that variation of local and reflex controls have on peripheral blood flow in terms of vasodilation, vasoconstriction, and baroreceptor activation.
2. Indicate the exchange that takes place at the capillaries of the lungs and body tissues, including fluids, nutrients, wastes, gases, and plasma proteins.
3. For each of the following elements, specify the effects of change on the fluid exchange throughout the capillaries in the lungs and body tissues: capillary hydrostatic pressure, interstitial hydrostatic pressure, plasma protein concentrations, and interstitial fluid protein concentrations.
4. List which materials are dependent on fluid flow for their transportation.
5. Specify the effects of malfunctions of the lymphatic system.

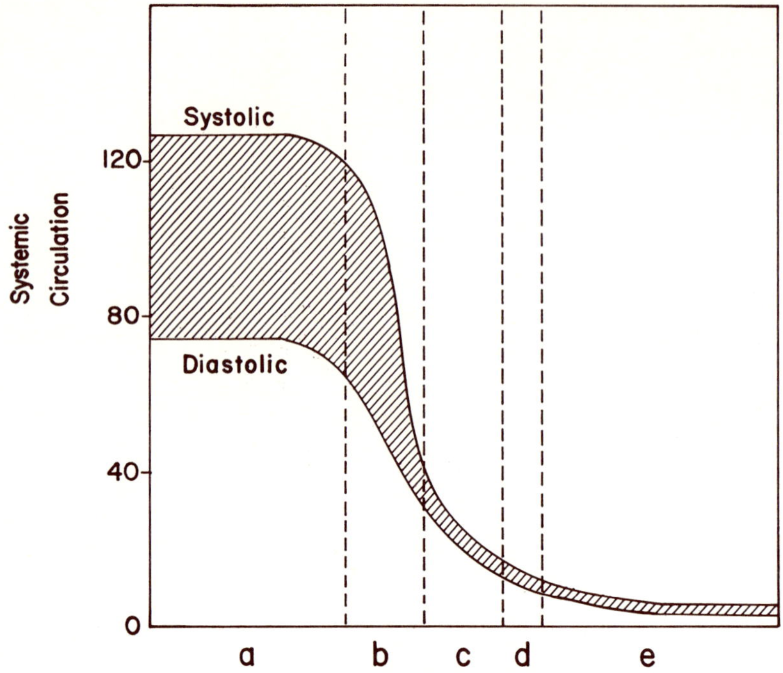

Fig. W-31 Pressure variation in the vascular system.

Reading Assignment

Chap. 9, pp. 246–263. Reread, concentrating on the functioning of the vessels.

Exercises

Part I

Directions: Label each section (*a* through *e*) of the accompanying graph (Fig. W-31), according to where the indicated pressure is located in the circulatory system. Use arteries, veins, arterioles, venules, and capillaries as labels. (Fig. 9-39, p. 260.)

a ______________________ *b* ______________________

c ______________________ *d* ______________________

e ______________________

Part II

Directions: Indicate by placing arrows on the appropriate lines in Fig. W-32 whether the materials are diffusing into or out of a normal capillary. (Fig. 9-37, pp. 256–257.)

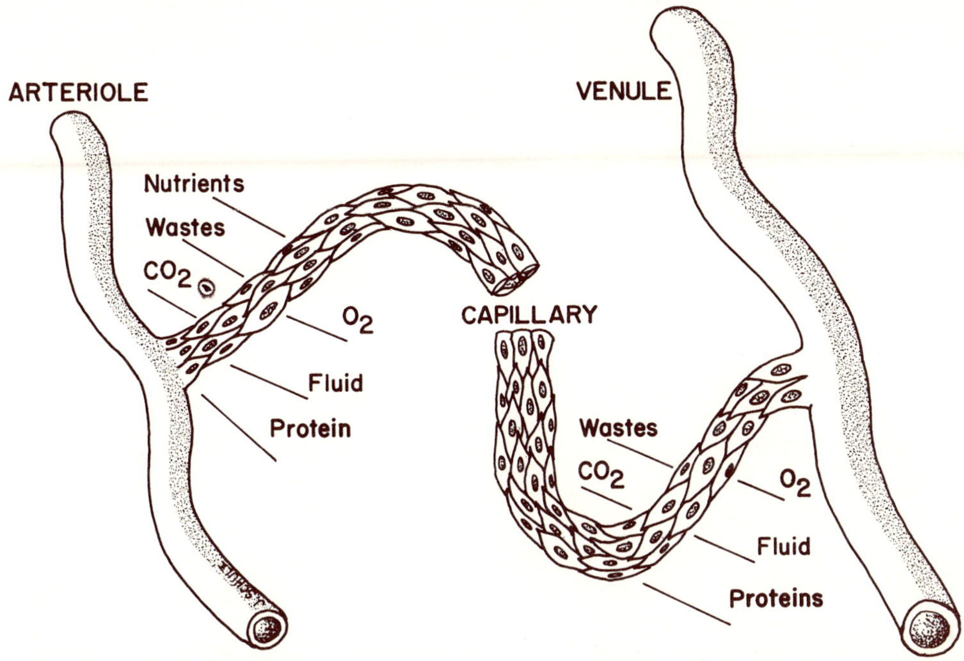

Fig. W-32 Capillary exchange.

Part III

Directions: Answer the following question. How would increased metabolic demands in the tissues served by the capillary in Part II change the diffusion of materials? *(256–260)*

Self-Test

Part I

Directions: Circle T for true and F for false. (Assume a normal capillary bed.)

T F 1. Blood pressure remains constant in the capillary beds.

T F 2. The difference between plasma and interstitial water concentration causes fluid to flow into the capillaries at the arteriolar ends.

T F 3. The high permeability of capillaries to proteins provides the osmotic gradient necessary to cause fluid to flow into the capillaries.

T F 4. Decreasing diameter of veins tends to increase venous blood pressure and increase blood return to the heart.

Part II

Directions: See the chart at the top of p. 88. Check in the appropriate spaces which of the four effects can be produced by each mechanism listed on the left.

	Effects			
	Dilation	Constriction	Decreased Flow	Increased Flow
Hormonal control				
Local control				
Reflex control				

Part III

Directions: Circle the correct answer(s).

1. The return of protein to the plasma by the lymphatics helps prevent edema by

   a maintaining protein concentration gradient at capillaries.
   b removing ultrafiltered fluid from tissue.
   c maintaining hydrostatic pressure in capillaries.

2. Most postganglionic sympathetic nerves release

   a epinephrine. *b* norepinephrine.
   c acetylcholine. *d* histamine.

3. Control of sympathetic nerve activity causes vascular smooth muscle to

   a contract. *b* relax.
   c both of the above. *d* remain the same.

4. Movement of nutrients and metabolic wastes through the capillary walls depends on

   a diffusion, primarily. *b* bulk flow, primarily.
   c neither diffusion nor bulk flow.

5. A blockage of a lymph vessel may cause

   a swelling of a limb (edema).
   b increased interstitial water concentration.
   c decreased interstitial protein concentration.

Part IV

Directions: Indicate whether ultrafiltration tends to increase or decrease in the following situations.

	Increase	Decrease
1. Capillary hydrostatic pressure rises.	______	______
2. Interstitial hydrostatic pressure drops.	______	______
3. Plasma protein concentration rises.	______	______
4. Interstitial fluid protein concentration drops.	______	______

Module VI: Integration of Cardiovascular Function

Objectives

Upon completion of this module, the student will be able to:

1. Indicate, by using the variables in the equation $F = \Delta P/R$ (F = flow, ΔP = pressure difference, R = resistance), the results of changes of any one variable on the others, in parts or all of the system, and relate this equation to cardiac output, arterial pressure, and total peripheral resistance.
2. Define the *total peripheral resistance* (TPR) and identify the relative importance of the different vessels. Note that the TPR excludes the resistance of the pulmonary circulation. *(266)*
3. Indicate the interaction of the parts of medullary cardiovascular center (MCVC), including the receptors, heart, arterioles, and veins. Indicate the mechanism of action for each part.
4. Locate in the body, by diagram or description, the carotid sinus, arch of the aorta, and medullary cardiovascular center (MCVC).
5. Distinguish between sensor and effector mechanisms in cardiovascular integration.
6. Outline the components of the baroreceptor reflex.

Reading Assignment

Chap. 9, pp. 263–271.

Exercises

Part I

Directions: Indicate with an arrow—($\uparrow$) for an increase, ($\downarrow$) for a decrease—the appropriate responses of each of the following to a decreased or increased rate of carotid sinus nerve impulses (Fig. 9-51, p. 271).

If the rate of carotid sinus nerve impulses were to:	Decrease	Increase
1. Heart rate would	______	______
2. Parasympathetic nerve impulse would	______	______
3. Peripheral resistance would	______	______
4. CO (cardiac output) would	______	______

Part II

Directions: Complete the following chart by indicating little or no change (↔), an increase (↑), or a decrease (↓) in each division of the autonomic nervous system (ANS) (Fig. 9-51 and 9-52, pp. 271–272).

	Division of ANS	
	↑ Parasympathetic	↑ Sympathetic
HR (heart rate)		
Total peripheral resistance		
CO (cardiac output)		
Blood flow to viscera		

Self-Test

Part I

Directions: Circle T for true and F for false.

T F 1. If one organ receives more blood through reduced arteriolar resistance, all other organs will receive less blood.

T F 2. Hyperemia is the dilation of arterioles in response to increased blood pressure.

T F 3. Arterial blood pressure tends to decrease in response to increasing arteriolar diameter.

T F 4. The carotid sinus nerves begin firing faster when the blood pressure drops below normal arterial pressure.

T F 5. Changes in length of the vasculature do not compensate for varied blood pressure needs.

T F 6. The total peripheral resistance is determined by the diameter of systemic arterioles in the body.

Part II

Directions: Write the number of the appropriate label in the correct location on Fig. W-33.

1. carotid sinus
2. arch of aorta
3. medullary cardiovascular center (MCVC)

Part III

Directions: Indicate with an arrow—(↑) for an increase, (↓) for a decrease—the appropriate responses of each of the following to a decreased or increased rate of carotid sinus nerve impulses.

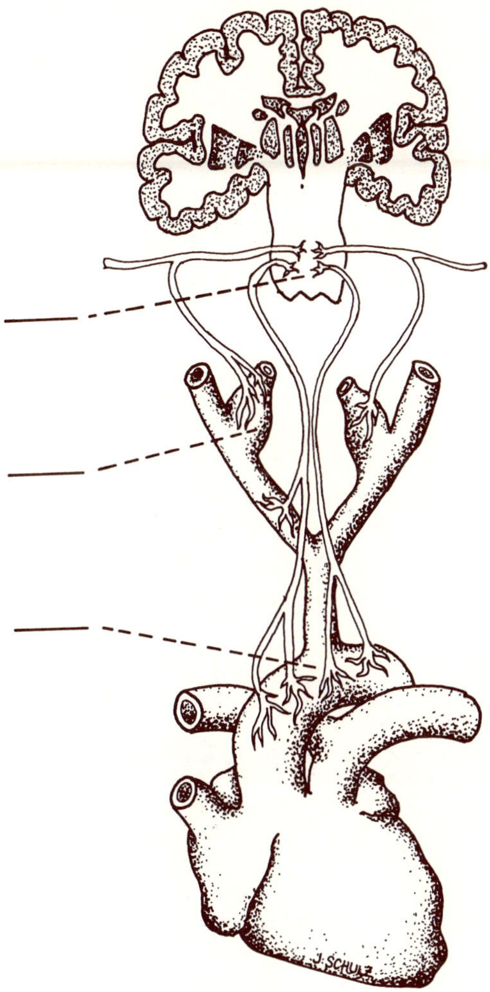

Fig. W-33

If the rate of carotid sinus nerve impulses were to:	Decrease	Increase
1. Heart rate would	______	______
2. Parasympathetic nerve impulse would	______	______
3. Peripheral resistance would	______	______
4. CO (cardiac output) would	______	______

Part IV

Directions: Complete the chart on p. 92 by indicating little or no change (↔), an increase (↑), or a decrease (↓) in each division of the autonomic nervous system (ANS).

	Division of ANS	
	↑ Parasympathetic	↑ Sympathetic
HR (heart rate)		
Total peripheral resistance		
CO (cardiac output)		
Blood flow to viscera		

Module VII: Cardiovascular Patterns in Health and Disease

Objectives

Upon completion of this module, the student will be able to:

1. Specify the compensatory mechanism used by the body to restore arterial pressure in hemorrhage, hypotension, and upright posture.
2. Identify shock in its various stages and specify the treatments.
3. Identify the general symptoms and causes of, and usual treatments for, hypertension, heart failure, arteriosclerosis, myocardial infarction, angina pectoris, valvular disease, and stroke.

Reading Assignment

Chap. 9, pp. 271–282.

Supplementary Materials

Murmurs during heartbeat can be classified according to the involved valve, as well as according to the time the murmur occurs. The chart below indicates the usual immediate cause of such murmurs.

Murmurs	Systole	Diastole
Aortic or pulmonary valves	Stenosis	Insufficiency
A-V valves	Insufficiency	Stenosis

Stenosis: a narrowing of one of the cardiac valves, resulting in turbulence.
Insufficiency: defective closure of a cardiac valve, resulting in leakage.

Exercises

Part I

Directions: On Fig. W-34, indicate with an arrow—(↑) for an increase, (↓) for a decrease—the change in each factor following hemorrhage (Fig. 9-53, p. 273).

Part II

Directions: Complete the following items in the space provided (Fig. 9-54, p. 275).

Little Violet Tinkwell just sat down in a dental-office waiting room. Little Violet is obviously uptight about what is going to happen to her in the next hour. She is definitely not looking well.

1. Her pallor is caused by ______________________________.
2. Her arterial blood pressure is ______________________________.

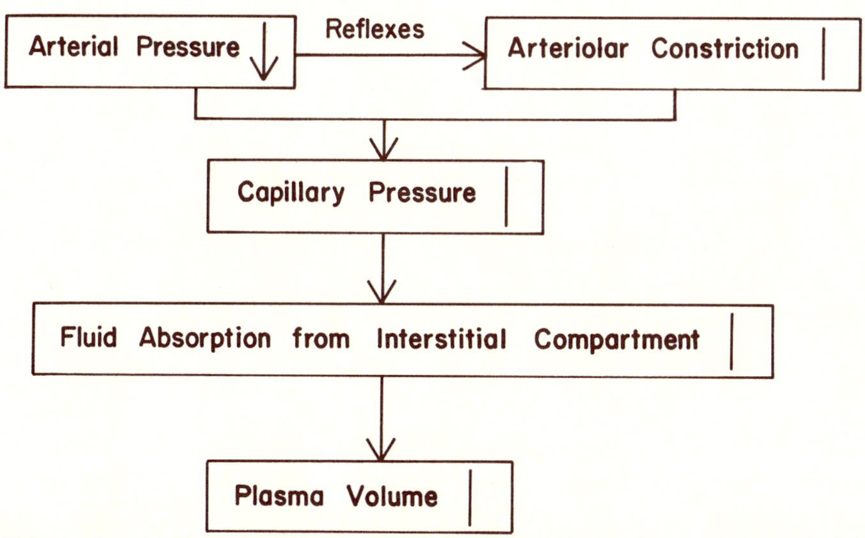

Fig. W-34 Cardiovascular pattern following hemorrhage.

3. The sympathetic activity from the medullary cardiovascular center is

   a increased ________

   b decreased ________

   while parasympathetic activity is

   c increased ________.

   d decreased ________.

4. Ms. Prissy Shiner, the faithful assistant, has an early lunch date. She stands Little Violet up and rushes her into the operating area. Little Violet, predictably, falls flat on her face. What happened to Little Violet's circulation that caused her to faint?

5. Since Mr. Tinkwell is a notorious attorney, it is advisable to treat Little Violet with care. What should you do to bring wilted Violet around? *(271–275)*

Self-Test

Part I

Directions: Circle the correct answer(s).

1. The direct effect(s) of hemorrhage before reflex adjustments occur is that

   a stroke volume increases. *b* heart rate increases.
   c cardiac output decreases.

2. Five minutes after hemorrhage stops

   a arterial pressure is above normal.
   b heart rate has increased.
   c erythrocyte volume is higher than normal.

3. Hypotension brought on by extreme emotion is caused by decreased

   a sympathetic activity from the MCVC.
   b parasympathetic activity from the MCVC.
   c arteriolar resistance.

4. The muscles of the legs help compensate for the effects of standing by

   a compressing the veins.
   b increasing hydrostatic pressure in capillaries.
   c forcing the blood through the veins.

5. During hemorrhage the water-concentration difference between capillaries and interstitial fluids is maintained due to the rapid synthesis of new plasma protein by the liver.

   a The statement above is true.
   b The statement above is false.
   c There is no basis for decision.

Part II

Directions: Circle the correct answer(s).

1. Accumulation of fluid in the lungs can result from

   a failure of left ventricle.
   b constriction of pulmonary arterioles.
   c dilation of pulmonary arterioles.
   d angina pectoris.

Module I:
Anatomy of the Respiratory System

Module II:
Mechanics of the Respiratory System

Module III:
Transport of Gas in the Body

Module IV:
Control of Respiration; Red Blood Cell Production

CHAPTER 10 RESPIRATION

Module I: Anatomy of the Respiratory System

Objectives

Upon completion of this module, the student will be able to:

1. Define *respiration, respiratory system, ventilation, inspiration,* and *expiration.*
2. Label the following structures on a diagram of the respiratory system and identify the function of each: esophagus, larynx, pharynx, trachea, bronchi, diaphragm, pleura, alveolus, bronchiole, alveolar duct, vocal cords, and glottis.
3. Identify three characteristics and/or functions of the cilia.
4. Identify the process by which gases are exchanged at the alveoli and at the tissues.

Reading Assignment

Chap. 10, pp. 283–287, and Chap. 12, pp. 361–362 (section on swallowing).

Exercises

Directions: In Fig. W-35 (p. 98), write in the names of the structures you know. Check your answers with the figures in the reading assignment, pp. 284–285.

Self-Test

Part I

Directions: Complete the following items in the space provided.

1. Those structures that are concerned with the exchange of gas between the blood and the external environment are called, collectively, the

   ______________________________.

2. The exchange of air between the atmosphere and the alveoli is called

   ______________________________.

3. The exchange of gas between the cells of the body and the external environment is

   ____.

Part II

Directions: Label the indicated structures in Fig. W-36 (p. 99).

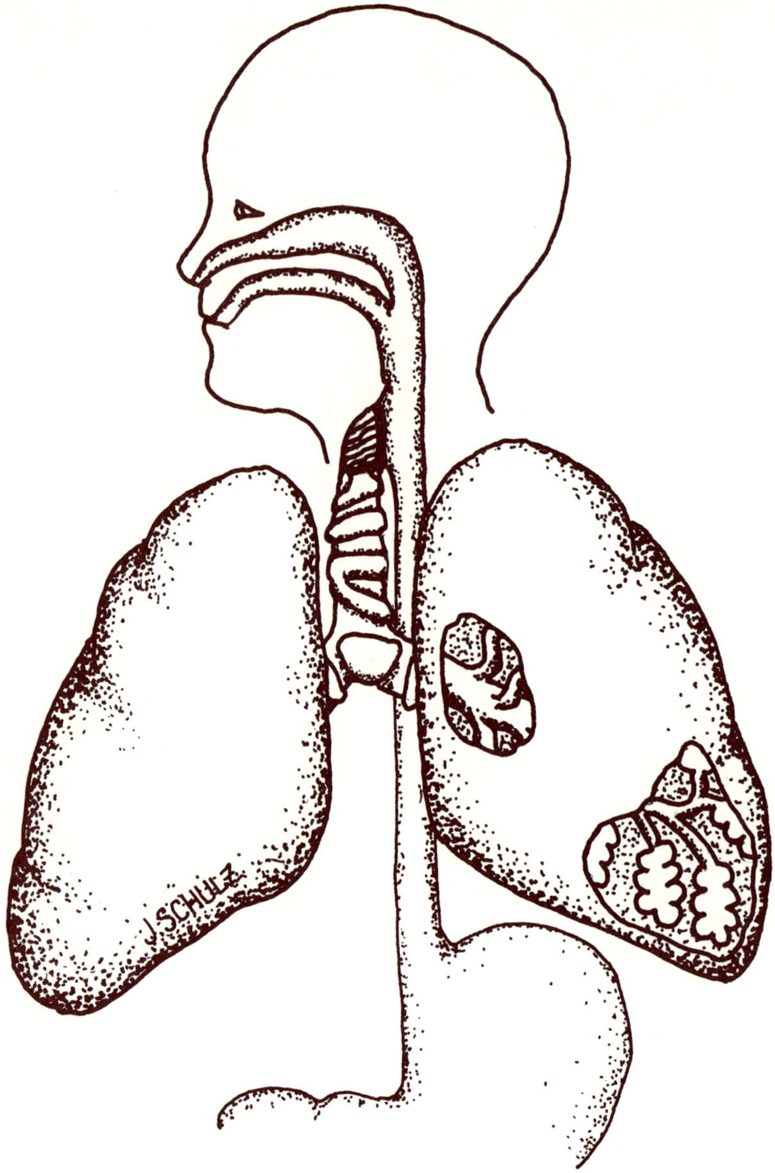

Fig. W-35

Part III

Directions: Circle T for true and F for false.

T F 1. The cilia are found in the pleura, near the alveoli.
T F 2. The cilia are hairlike projections on the epithelial linings of the pharynx.
T F 3. The cilia help move mucus along the air passages toward the larynx.
T F 4. The alveoli are filled with intrapleural fluid.
T F 5. The cilia provide a defense against infection by keeping the air passages clean.

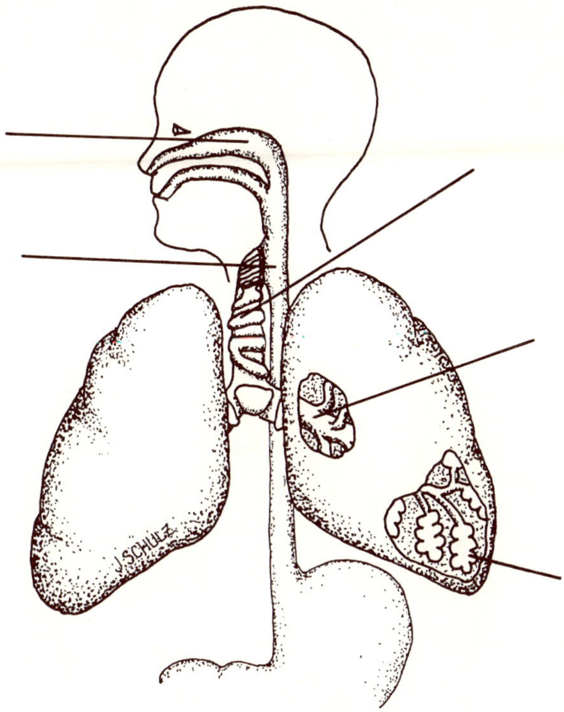

Fig. W-36

Part IV

Directions: Circle the correct answer(s).

1. Oxygen and carbon dioxide are exchanged between alveolar air and the capillaries, and between the blood and the tissues, through a process called:

   a bulk flow   *b* ingestion
   c diffusion   *d* confusion

Module II: Mechanics of the Respiratory System

Objectives

Upon completion of this module, the student will be able to:

1. Identify the effects of pressure on the bulk flow of air between the alveoli and the atmosphere by writing the equation for bulk flow and identifying each variable.
2. Compare intrapleural and intrathoracic pressure.
3. List the steps in inspiration and expiration. (See Fig. 10-9, p. 289.)
4. List three factors which determine the amount of resistance to air flow in the lungs.
5. Describe the effect of physical and nervous factors on airway resistance.
6. Identify the local effects of increased and decreased concentrations of carbon dioxide on the bronchioles.
7. Identify the local effects of increased and decreased concentrations of oxygen on the pulmonary arterioles.
8. Identify (see Fig. W-37 in supplementary materials), and give the approximate normal value of, and describe the measurement of tidal volume, inspiratory reserve volume, expiratory reserve volume, residual volume, total lung volume, inspiratory capacity, vital capacity, and total lung capacity (same as total lung volume).
9. Given the appropriate data, calculate the total pulmonary ventilation per minute.
10. Distinguish between minute ventilatory volume and alveolar ventilation, and anatomic dead space and alveolar dead space.
11. Identify factors which help determine the "work of breathing."
12. Define *pneumothorax, vital capacity, pulmonary surfactant, asthma, compliance of respiratory system, lung,* and *thoracic cage.*

Reading Assignment

Chap. 10, pp. 287–295.

Supplementary Materials

The following material will define *compliance* of the respiratory system, lung, and thoracic cage.

The "stretchability" of a system is called its compliance. For the respiratory system

$$\frac{1}{\text{Compliance (system)}} = \frac{1}{\text{compliance (lung)}} + \frac{1}{\text{compliance (thoracic cage)}}$$

Each of these compliances is defined by:

$$\text{Compliance} = \frac{\text{change in volume}}{\text{change in pressure}}$$

A soft, flabby balloon has a high compliance (i.e., is very easily stretched) and a large volume change is produced by a small pressure change. If the compliance decreases, then

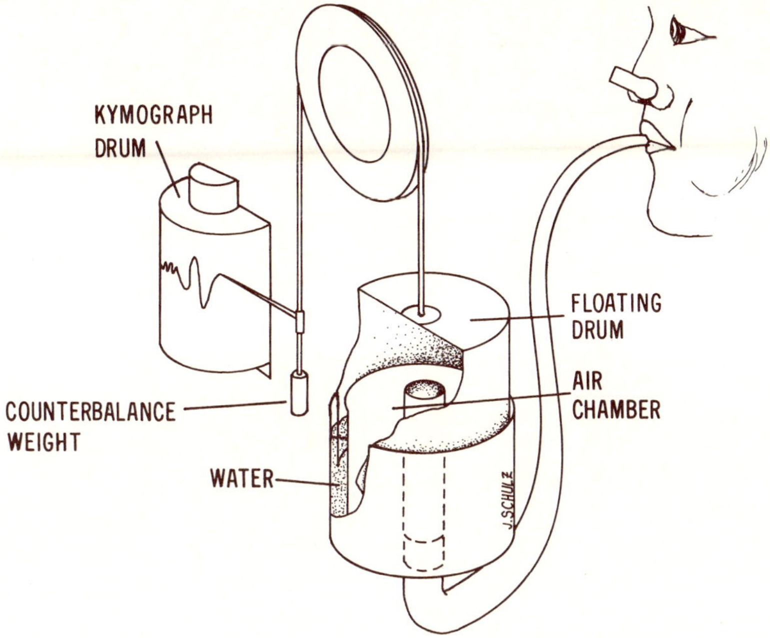

Fig. W-37

greater pressure is required to produce the same volume change. Numerous disease states are characterized by decreased compliance.

Figure W-37 is a schematic diagram of a laboratory spirometer, a device used to measure lung volume. The subject breathes through a tube, causing the floating drum to move up and down. These movements cause deflections in the pen which traces the respiratory movements on the kymograph drum. Figure W-38 represents an idealized tracing of the various respiratory volumes described in the text.

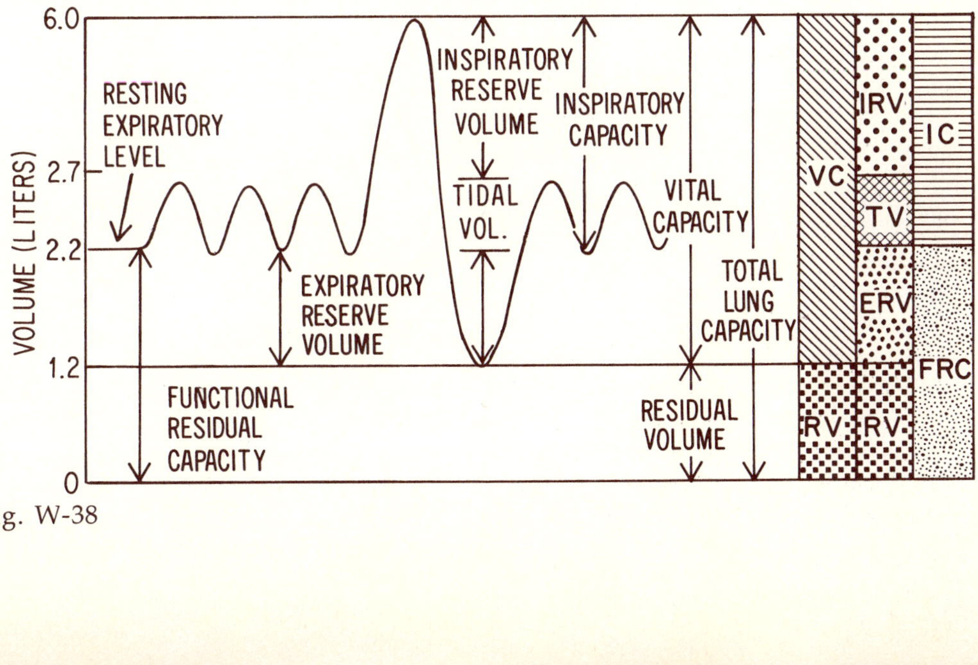

Fig. W-38

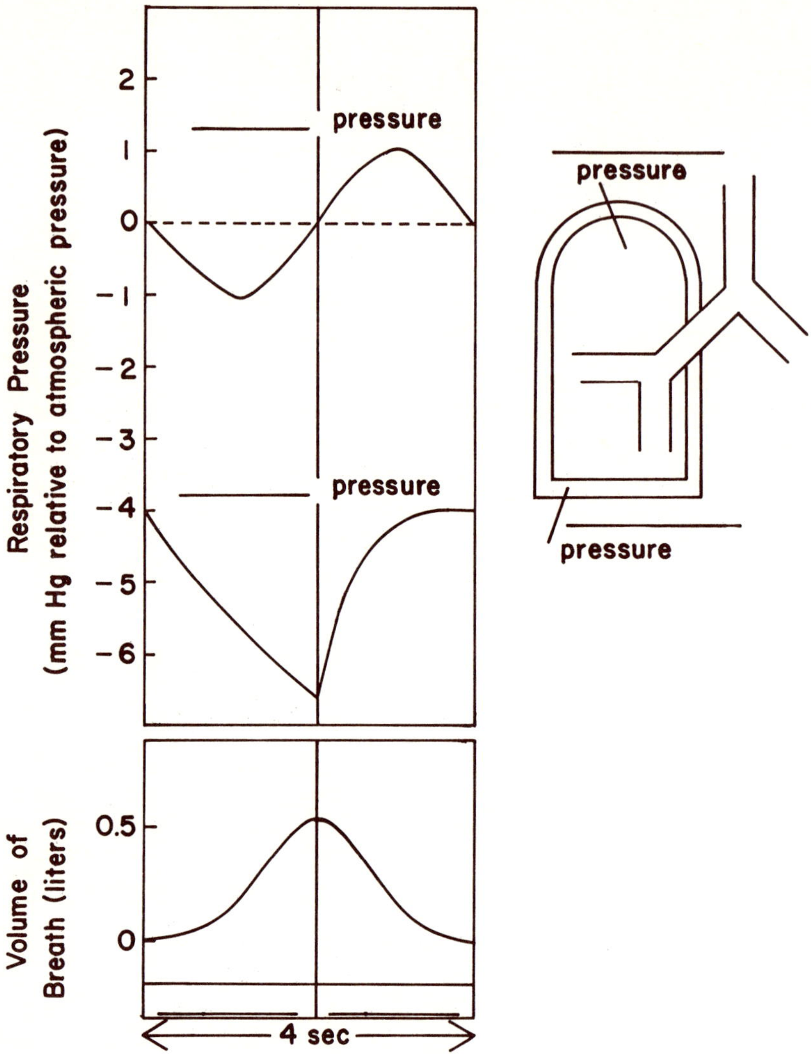

Fig. W-39 Pressure.

Exercises

Part I

Directions: Fill in the labels on Fig. W-39, indicating the specific types of pressure. You can check your answers against Fig. 10-9, p. 289.

Part II

Directions: Complete Charts 1 and 2 to calculate alveolar ventilation. Use 150 ml as the volume for the dead-space volume. In Chart 2 use the frequency values given in Chart 1 to calculate the dead-space ventilation. You can check your calculations for entries A, C, and D with Table 10-2, p. 294.

Chart 1

Subject	Tidal Volume, (ml/breath)	×	Frequency (breath/min)	=	Total Pulmonary Ventilation (ml/min)
A	150	×	40	=	______
B	250	×	24	=	______
C	500	×	12	=	______
D	1000	×	6	=	______

In Chart 2 use the values calculated in Chart 1 for the total pulmonary ventilation for subjects A through D. Again, use 150 ml as the dead-space value and the frequencies of respiration provided above.

Chart 2

Subject	Total Pulmonary Ventilation	−	Dead-Space Ventilation (dead-space vol. × frequency, ml/breath × breath/min)	=	Alveolar Ventilation
	ml/min	−	ml/min	=	ml/min
A	______		______	=	0
B	6000	−	(150) × (24)	=	______
C	______	−	______	=	4200
D	______	−	900	=	5100

Part III

Directions: Label the lung volumes on Fig. W-40. Check your answers with Fig. 10-14, p. 293.

Part IV

Directions: This exercise will take you through the steps in respiration. Answer the questions in order, as many depend on previous responses. Circle the correct answer(s) or fill in the spaces.

1. No air is flowing, all respiratory muscles are relaxed. The subject is in the stage
   a of inspiration.
   b at the end of inspiration prior to expiration.
   c of expiration.
   d at the end of expiration and prior to inspiration. *(289)*

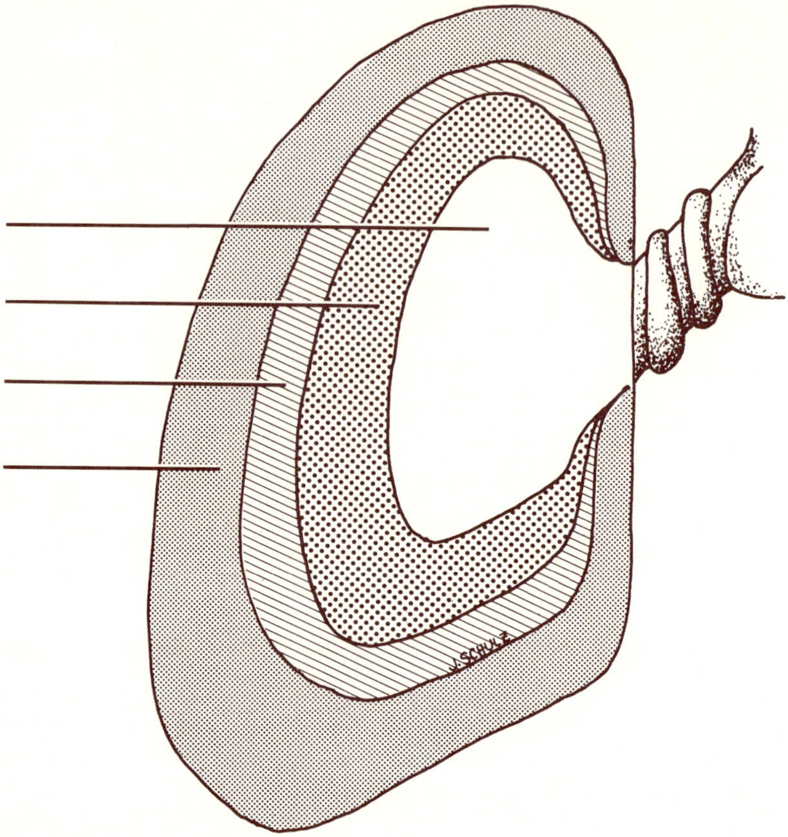

Fig. W-40 Lung volumes.

2. The intrapleural pressure at rest is

   a atmospheric. *b* subatmospheric.
   c greater than atmospheric. (287)

3. The intraalveolar pressure at rest is

   a atmospheric. *b* subatmospheric.
   c greater than atmospheric. (289)

4. At this point, inspiration is initiated. The *first* step is

   a contraction of the alveoli.
   b simultaneous contraction of the diaphragm and intercostal muscles causing an enlargement of the chest cavity.
   c an increase in intrapleural pressure. (289)

5. When the intrapleural pressure becomes even more subatmospheric, what effect does it have on the intraalveolar pressure? ____________________ (289)

6. The result of the dropping of intraalveolar pressure below atmospheric pressure is ____________________. (289)

7. At the end of inspiration, the intraalveolar pressure is

_____________________. (289)

8. The intrapleural pressure is _____________________. (289)

9. The expiration is initiated by relaxation of what muscle(s)? _____________________

_____________________ (289)

10. What effect does the decrease in size of the thoracic cavity have on the intrapleural pressure? _____________________

On the intraalveolar pressure? _____________________

_____________________ (289)

11. What is the net result of the increase in intrapleural and intraalveolar pressure?

_____________________ (289)

Self-Test

Part I

Directions: Write in the term or phrase that describes each definition or example below.

1. Air in the intrapleural space _____________________.
2. Pressure that is always subatmospheric during normal breathing

   _____________________.
3. Movement of air into or out of the lungs _____________________.
4. Total amount of air that can be moved in and out during a single breath

   _____________________.
5. Volume of air in lungs after a forceful expiration

   _____________________.
6. Volume of air breathed into or out of the lungs in a normal breath

   _____________________.
7. Volume of air that can be breathed out after a single expiration

   _____________________.
8. Volume of air that can be breathed in after a normal inspiration

   _____________________.
9. Sum of tidal, inspiratory reserve, and expiratory reserve volumes

   _____________________.
10. The phospholipid lining of the alveoli _____________________.
11. Tidal volume times the number of respirations per minute is called

    _____________________.
12. The normal value for _____________________ dead space is 150 ml.

13. Alveolar ventilation is calculated as the frequency of breathing times (tidal volume minus ____________________).
14. If your inspiratory reserve volume is 300 ml, your expiratory reserve volume is 400 ml, and your vital capacity is 1800 ml, how much air do you normally breathe in or out in a single breath while resting? ____________________.

Part II

Directions: Circle the correct answer(s).

1. Intrathoracic pressure is

   a greater than
   b less than
   c synonymous with intrapleural pressure

2. The change in intrapleural pressure from −4 mmHg to −8 mmHg during inspiration is due to the

   a expansion of the thoracic cage.
   b compression of the abdomen.
   c pumping action of the larynx.
   d compression of the thoracic cage.

3. Inspiration is normally a(n) (active, passive) process and expiration is normally a(n) (active, passive) process.
4. The volume of air flow to the alveoli is increased when there is an increase in

   a resistance in the airway.
   b the pressure gradient between atmosphere and the alveoli.
   c the size of the diameters of the airways.
   d the length of the airways.

Part III

Directions: Complete the following items in the space provided.

1. Smooth muscles of the bronchioles are especially sensitive to local concentrations of ____________________; smooth muscles of the pulmonary arterioles are especially sensitive to local concentrations of ____________________.
2. The volume of air still remaining in the lungs after a maximal expiration is the ____________________; its approximate normal value is ____________________ ml.
3. The amount of air which can be inspired or expired beyond the resting tidal volume is the inspiratory or expiratory ____________________. The normal volumes, respectively, are about ________ ml and ________ ml.

4. The volume of air entering or leaving the lungs in a single breath is the

______________________________; its normal, resting volume is about

________ ml.

5. List the volumes whose sum is the vital capacity.

6. Directions: Complete Charts 1 and 2 to calculate alveolar ventilation. Use 150 ml as the volume for the dead-space volume. In Chart 2 use the frequency values given in Chart I to calculate the dead-space ventilation.

Chart 1

Subject	Tidal Volume (ml/breath)	×	Frequency (breaths/min)	=	Total Pulmonary Ventilation (ml/min)
A	150	×	40	=	________
B	250	×	24	=	________
C	500	×	12	=	________
D	1000	×	6	=	________

In Chart 2 use the values calculated in Chart 1 for the total pulmonary ventilation for subjects A through D. Again, use 150 ml as the dead-space volume and the frequencies of respiration provided above.

Chart 2

Subject	Total Pulmonary Ventilation ml/min	–	Dead-Space Ventilation (dead-space vol. × frequency, ml/breath × breaths/min) ml/min	=	Alveolar Ventilation ml/min
A					0
B	6000	–	(150) × (24)	=	
C		–		=	4200
D		–	900	=	5100

Part IV

Directions: Circle T for true and F for false.

T F 1. The conducting airways cannot exchange gas, and their volume is called the alveolar dead space.

T F 2. Two factors closely related to the "work of breathing" are the stretchability of the lungs and the amount of airway resistance.

T F 3. Pneumothorax aids in alveolar ventilation.

T F 4. Asthma causes a dilation of the airways and an increase in the anatomic dead space.

Module III: Transport of Gas in the Body

Objectives

Upon completion of this module, the student will be able to:

1. Define *respiratory quotient* (RQ) and state, as examples, the RQs of glucose and fat.
2. List the steps in the exchange of oxygen and carbon dioxide between the atmosphere and the lungs, and between the blood and tissues.
3. Define *passive diffusion, gas pressure,* and *partial pressure of gas.*
4. List two factors which determine the amount of gas which can be dissolved in a liquid.
5. Indicate the reasons that the partial pressures of expired air are different from the partial pressures of atmospheric air and alveolar air, and that there is little variation in the partial pressures of oxygen and carbon dioxide in the alveoli.
6. Specify the two forms in which oxygen is carried in the blood with an approximate percentage carried in each form.
7. Define *hemoglobin, oxyhemoglobin, reduced hemoglobin,* and *dissolved blood gases,* and describe the role of each in the transport of gas in the blood.
8. State the effects on the oxygen dissociation curve of changes in the acidity of the blood (see Supplementary Materials).
9. State the effects on the oxygen dissociation curve of changes in the temperature of the blood.
10. Compare hemoglobin and myoglobin in composition, location, dissociation curve, and function.
11. List the three forms in which carbon dioxide is carried in the body with the approximate percentage carried in each form.

12. Name the function served by carbonic anhydrase and the site of action within the blood.
13. Name the two end products of the ionization of carbonic acid.
14. Name at least two conditions which impair the diffusion of gases through the alveoli.

Reading Assignment

Chap. 10, pp. 295–306.

Supplementary Materials

The loading of CO_2 and the unloading of O_2 in the body tissues facilitate one another. As the PCO_2 in the capillaries increases (pH ↓), oxygen unloading from hemoglobin is facilitated. This is known as the Bohr effect. See Fig. 10-18, p. 300.

Exercises

Part I

Directions: Complete the following items in the space provided.

1. Assume that your respiratory system produces eight molecules of carbon dioxide for every ten molecules of oxygen consumed. What is your respiratory quotient?

   ________________ What would be the RQ if pure glucose were used for energy? ________________ If pure fat were used?

   ________________ *(296)*

2. Atmospheric pressure at sea level is 760 mmHg. If air contains 21 percent oxygen, what is the partial pressure of oxygen (PO_2) at sea level?

   ________________ *(298)*

3. Refer to Fig. 10-17, p. 298, to answer these questions.

   a PO_2 is highest in the ________________.

   b Except for the cells, PO_2 is lowest in the ________________.

   c Except for the cells, PCO_2 is highest in the ________________.

   d PCO_2 is lowest in the ________________.

   e In alveolar air, PCO_2 is (>, =, <) the PCO_2 of expired air. ________

   f In alveolar air, PO_2 is (>, =, <) the PO_2 of expired air. ________

4. List in order five steps in carbon dioxide exchange between cells and alveoli.

   a ________________ *b* ________________

   c ________________ *d* ________________

   e ________________ *(305)*

5. Oxygen in the blood can be carried in two ways.

   a combined with hemoglobin
   b dissolved in the blood

   The percentage saturation refers to which of these? ________ *(299)*

6. Refer to the text if necessary and enter the approximate percentages of carbon dioxide beside each of the following entries.

   physically dissolved ________

   HCO_3^- ________

   $HbCO_2$ ________ *(305)*

7. The percentage saturation is affected by

   a the size of the individual. *b* temperature.
   c acidity. *d* PO_2. *(302)*

Part II

Directions: Arrange these steps in order. Enter the number of the step (1, 2, etc.) in the space provided.

________ O_2 enters pulmonary capillaries.

________ O_2 leaves tissue capillaries.

________ O_2 crosses alveolar membrane.

________ O_2 crosses cell membrane.

________ O_2 is transported in the bloodstream. *(298)*

Self-Test

Part I

Directions: Complete the following items in the space provided.

1. Write the equation for the respiratory quotient (RQ).

   RQ = ________________________________.

2. What is the respiratory quotient for glucose? ________________________________.

   For fat? ________________________________.

3. The pressure of a gas is proportional to its ________________________________

   and ________________________________.

4. The movement of molecules from an area of high concentration to an area of low concentration usually occurs passively by ________________________________.

5. The amount of oxygen entering a liquid from a gas is a function of

   a ________________________________

   b ________________________________.

6. The partial pressures of gases vary by only a small amount in the alveoli. Briefly explain why this is so.

7. Name two forms in which oxygen is carried in the blood, and give the approximate percentage of oxygen carried in each form.

   a ____ ________%

   b ____ ________%

8. Name the three forms in which carbon dioxide is carried in the blood, and give the approximate percentage of carbon dioxide carried in each form.

   a ____ ________%

   b ____ ________%

   c ____ ________%

9. What catalyst facilitates the reaction:

   $CO_2 + H_2O \leftrightharpoons H_2CO_3$? ____.

10. What are the two end products of the ionization of carbonic acid?

    a ____

    b ____

11. Name two conditions which can impair the diffusion of gases into the blood.

    a ____

    b ____

Part II

Directions: Think back to Miss Truedale's algebra class. The symbols > (greater than) and < (less than) were used to show a relationship between two quantities. Insert the appropriate symbol between the values below.

1. PO_2 in inspired air ________ PO_2 in alveolar air.
2. PO_2 in alveolar air ________ PO_2 in pulmonary arteries and systemic veins.
3. PO_2 in tissues ________ PO_2 in pulmonary veins and systemic arteries.
4. PCO_2 in expired air ________ PCO_2 in alveolar air.
5. PCO_2 in alveolar air ________ PCO_2 in pulmonary arteries and systemic veins.
6. PCO_2 in tissues ________ PCO_2 in pulmonary veins and systemic arteries.

Part III

Directions: Put an M before statements true for myoglobin, and an H before statements true for hemoglobin.

1. ________ found in the muscles
2. ________ found in the erythrocytes
3. ________ an iron-containing protein
4. ________ a copper-containing protein

Module IV: Control of Respiration; Red Blood Cell Production

Objectives

Upon completion of this module, the student will be able to:

1. Identify two current theories (not necessarily incompatible) which account for the rhythmicity of breathing.
2. List the three sources of input to the medullary inspiratory neurons.
3. Name and locate the receptors for a low partial pressure of oxygen in the body.
4. Define *hypoxic, anemic, ischemic* and *histotoxic hypoxia,* and give examples of each.
5. Compare the effects of low partial pressures of oxygen and carbon dioxide on increasing the minute respiratory volume.
6. Identify the major points of the theory of hydrogen ion influence on respiration.
7. Identify characteristic changes in ventilation during exercise, and give the reasons that stimuli of PO_2, PCO_2, and H^+ do not adequately account for these changes.
8. Identify the steps in the "life cycle" of an erythrocyte.
9. Describe the roles of iron and vitamin B_{12} by specifying their major function, the site of control of balance, and the result of deficiency.
10. Define *erythropoiesis* and *erythropoietin.*
11. Specify the consequences of hyperventilation and hypoventilation.

Reading Assignment

Chap. 10, pp. 306–318.

Supplementary Materials

Definitions:

Eupnea: easy or normal respiration.
Hyperpnea: abnormal *increase* in the depth and rate of the respiratory movements.
Hypopnea: abnormal *decrease* in the depth and rate of the respiratory movements.
Apnea: the absence of respiratory movements.

Exercises

Part I

Directions: Complete the following items in the space provided.

1. So far as rhythm is concerned, the three major inputs to the medullary inspiratory neuron serve different functions. Write the source of input after each of these functions:

   a serves as a central relay station: tonic effect ______________________ *(307)*

   b initiates respiratory inhibition, either directly or through the pons

   ______________________ *(307)*

   c helps terminate discharge of inspiratory neuron; stimulates nerves to expiratory muscles ______________________ *(308)*

2. When one inhales carbon monoxide, the ventilatory rate does not increase significantly, even though death may ensue from oxygen lack. Why is it that the oxygen lack does not increase the breathing rate and depth? ______________________ *(310)*

3. A decrease in PO_2 causes increased ventilation by stimulation of what organs? ____________

   ______________________ *(310)*

4. Suppose you are performing an experiment in which the subject hyperventilates for 5 min. Then you ask him to breathe normally (this was 17 breaths/min before hyperventilation). What would you expect to happen to his breathing rate?

   ______________________ *(311)*

5. This erythrocyte, Sam, shown in Fig. W-41 (p. 114), was formed in the

   ______________________ of the body by the process of

   ______________________. Sam's life expectancy is

   ______________________. He will meet his end, and his little corpse

   will be consumed by a ______________________. A true-blue conservationist to the end, Sam will donate his remains to the body, especially the

   hemoglobin, which will be broken down to ______________________.
   Rest in peace, Sam. *(316–317)*

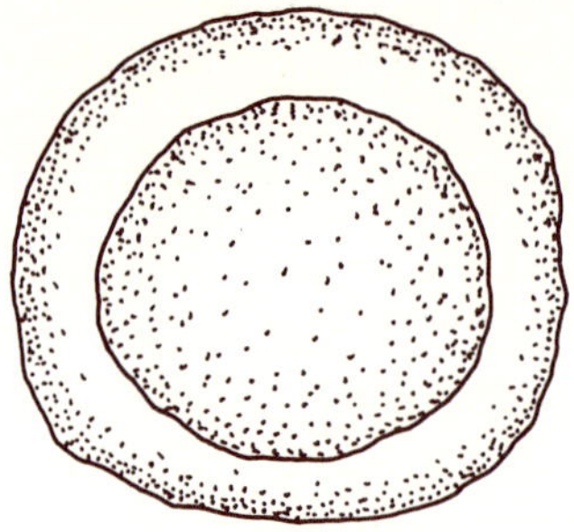

Fig. W-41

Part II

Directions: Circle the correct answer(s).

1. You ordinarily breathe in a rhythmical way. Which explanations below might explain the rhythmicity of breathing?

   a inherent automaticity and rhythmicity of inspiratory neurons
   b excitatory synaptic input to the inspiratory neurons
   c inputs by the proprioceptive neurons to the inspiratory neurons (*307*)

2. The experiment in Part I, question 4 could have been designed to investigate

   a the effect of increased PO_2 on breathing.
   b the effect of increased PCO_2 on breathing.
   c the usefulness of hyperventilation for competitive swimmers. (*311*)

3. When an individual is involved in heavy exercise, his alveolar ventilation is increased ten to twenty times. Which of the following are true of the heavy exercise?

   a Anatomic dead space decreases. (*293–294*)
   b Arterial PO_2 is drastically reduced. (*313*)
   c Excess hydrogen ions accumulate in the venous flow. (*314*)
   d The chemical changes in the blood do not fully explain the ventilation pattern. (*314*)

Self-Test

Part I

Directions: Circle the correct answer(s).

1. There remains some controversy about the factors causing the rhythmic firing of the inspiratory neurons in the brain stem. Your textbook supports which of the following views?

   a These neurons have an inherent automaticity and rhythmicity.
   b These neurons require excitatory synaptic input.
   c Both (*a*) and (*b*).
   d Neither (*a*) nor (*b*).

2. The medullary inspiratory neurons receive inputs from three *major* sources which are important in maintaining normal breathing rhythm. Which three of the following are the *major* sources?

   a reciprocal connections with the medullary expiratory neurons
   b connections with the thalamus
   c connections with the pons
   d carotid sinus and aortic arch
   e stretch receptors in the lungs

3. Which of the following conditions reduces the oxygen content of the blood without concurrently dropping the partial pressure of oxygen in the blood?

   a hypoxia *b* anemia
   c emphysema *d* carbon monoxide poisoning
   e asthma

4. The minute respiratory volume is most readily increased by a

   a low PO_2 in inspired air.
   b high PCO_2 in inspired air.

5. The concentration of H^+ in which of the following has the greatest influence on respiration?

   a tissues *b* blood *c* alveoli
   d cerebrospinal fluid *e* kidneys

6. Which of the following has been identified as the major variable contributing to the ventilation changes during exercise?

   a PCO_2 *b* H^+ concentration
   c temperature *d* PO_2
   e none of the above

Part II

Directions: Complete each of the items below in the space provided.

1. Two receptors for the partial pressure of oxygen are

   a ______________________________

   b ______________________________

2. Recent studies indicate that an increase in H^+ concentration (increases/decreases) ______________ the rate of inspiratory neuron firing, while the rate of firing is (increased/decreased) ______________ by a decreased H^+ concentration.

3. Breathing as rapidly and deeply as possible is called ______________.

4. Breathing slowly and shallowly as possible results in ______________.

5. A complete cessation of breathing (assuming it is for an excessively long period terminating in death) is called ______________.

Part III

Directions: These are statements about erythrocytes. Circle T for true and F for false.

T F 1. Erythrocytes are produced in the bone marrow, the liver, and the spleen.

T F 2. The average life-span of an erythrocyte is about 4 months.

T F 3. Erythrocytes are produced by a process called erythropoietin.

T F 4. Some of the raw materials required to produce erythrocytes are iron, vitamin B_{12}, folic acid, and amino acids.

T F 5. Bilirubin is the component of the hemoglobin molecule with which the oxygen actually combines.

T F 6. Iron balance is maintained by the kidneys, while vitamin B_{12} is dependent on dietary intake and its balance is maintained by the gastrointestinal system.

T F 7. The erythrocyte is frequently called an incomplete cell as it lacks a nucleus.

T F 8. While little is known about the hormone which stimulates the production of erythrocytes, it does increase in amount in response to a decreased delivery of oxygen to the tissues.

T F 9. When the erythrocyte dies, the large molecules are broken down by antibodies in the liver, spleen, bone marrow, and lymph nodes.

T F 10. The oxygen-carrying capacity of the erythrocytes is not significantly diminished by the aging of the cell.

Module I:
Regulation of the Internal Environment

Module II:
Basic Function of the Nephron and Micturition

Module III:
Regulation of the Renal Function, Part I

Module IV:
Regulation of the Renal Function, Part II

REGULATION OF WATER AND ELECTROLYTE BALANCE

CHAPTER 11

Module I: Regulation of the Internal Environment

Objectives

Upon completion of this module the student will be able to:

1. State the major function of the kidney as described in the reading using the concepts of balance, and internal and external exchanges.
2. Identify the following five major substances regulated by the kidney: H_2O, Na^+, Ca^{2+}, K^+, and H^+.
3. Given a diagram of the nephron and associated blood vessels label on the diagram the following items: glomerulus, Bowman's capsule, proximal tubule, loop of Henle, distal tubule, collecting duct, afferent arteriole, efferent arteriole, peritubular capillaries (see Fig. 11-3, p. 322); also indicate (using arrows) the direction of blood and urine flows.
4. Given a diagram of a sagittal section of the kidney, label the following items: cortex, medulla, renal pelvis, ureter, bladder, urethra, direction of urine flow (using arrows).

Reading Assignment

Chap. 11, pp. 319–322. Pay particular attention to figures and to Table 11-1.

Exercises

Label Figs. W-42 (p. 119) and W-43 (p. 120) as indicated. *(321–322)*

Self-Test

Part I

Directions: Answer the following questions in the space provided.

1. What is the major function of the kidney in the human body?

____

____

2. Identify five major substances regulated by the kidney.

a ______________________________

b ______________________________

c ______________________________

d ______________________________

e ______________________________

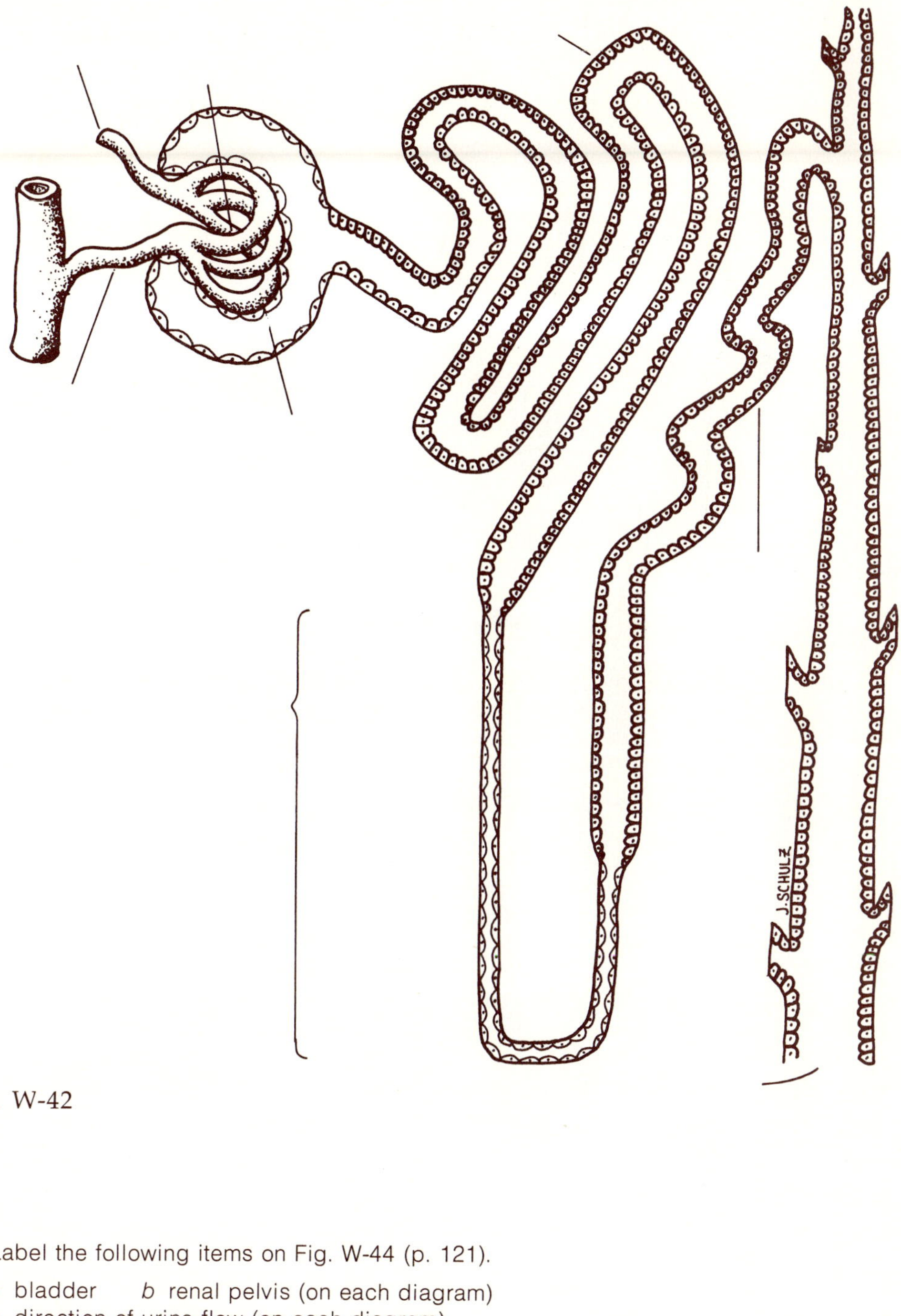

Fig. W-42

3. Label the following items on Fig. W-44 (p. 121).

   a bladder *b* renal pelvis (on each diagram)
   c direction of urine flow (on each diagram)
   d medulla *e* cortex *f* ureter

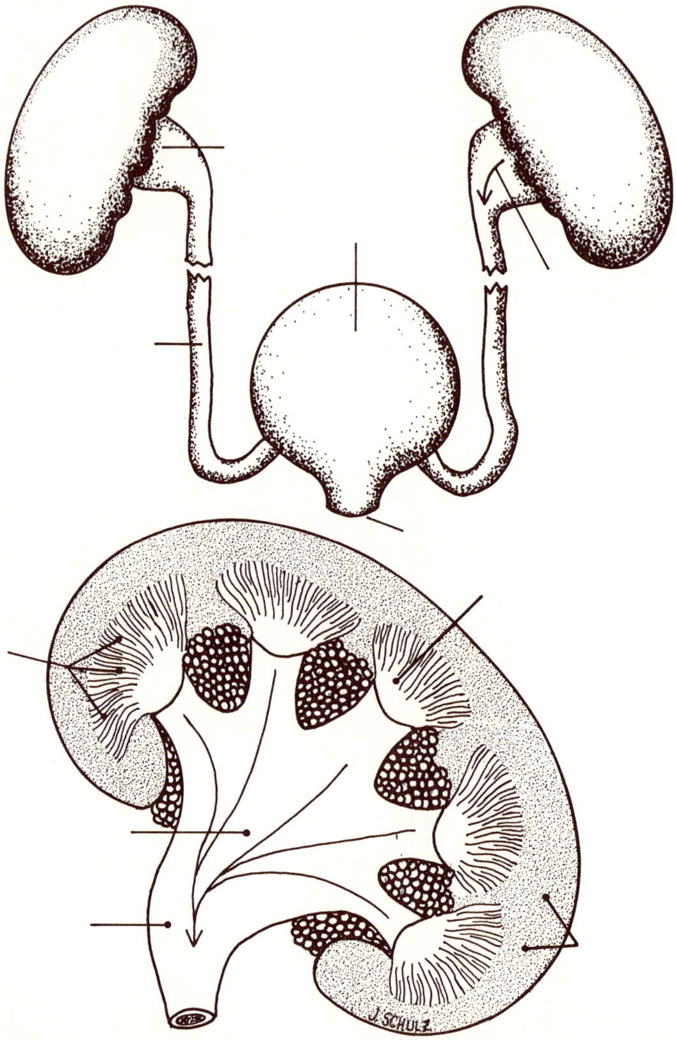

Fig. W-43 Structure of the urinary system.

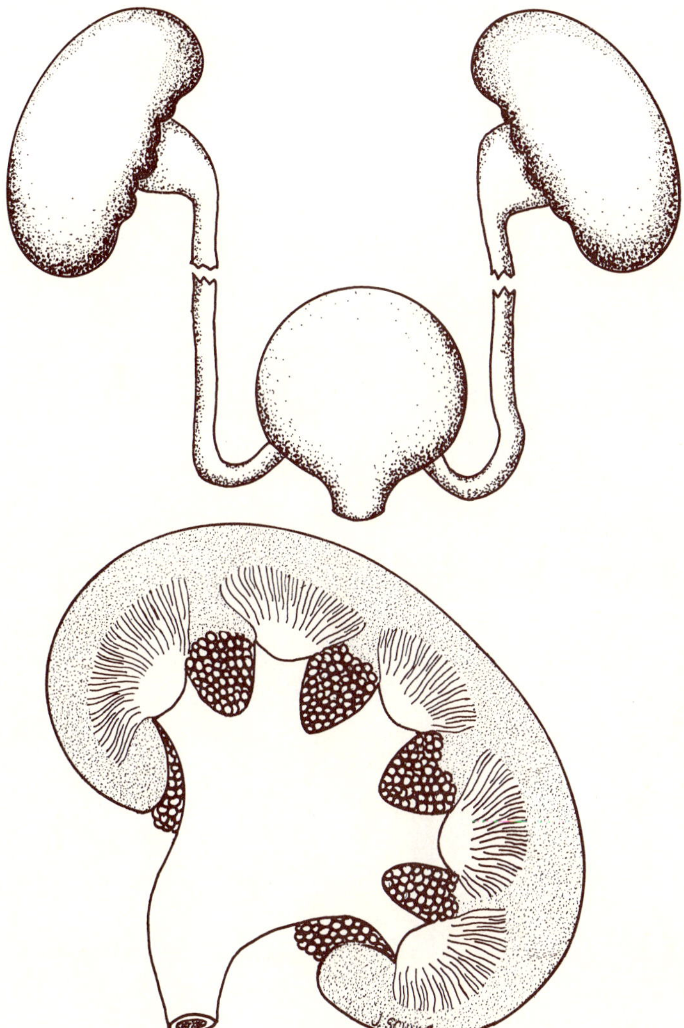

Fig. W-44 Structure of the urinary system.

Part II

Directions: Label the following items on Fig. W-45.

1. glomerulus
2. Bowman's capsule
3. proximal tubule
4. loop of Henle
5. distal tubule
6. collecting duct
7. afferent arteriole
8. efferent arteriole
9. direction of blood and urine flow (use arrows to indicate)

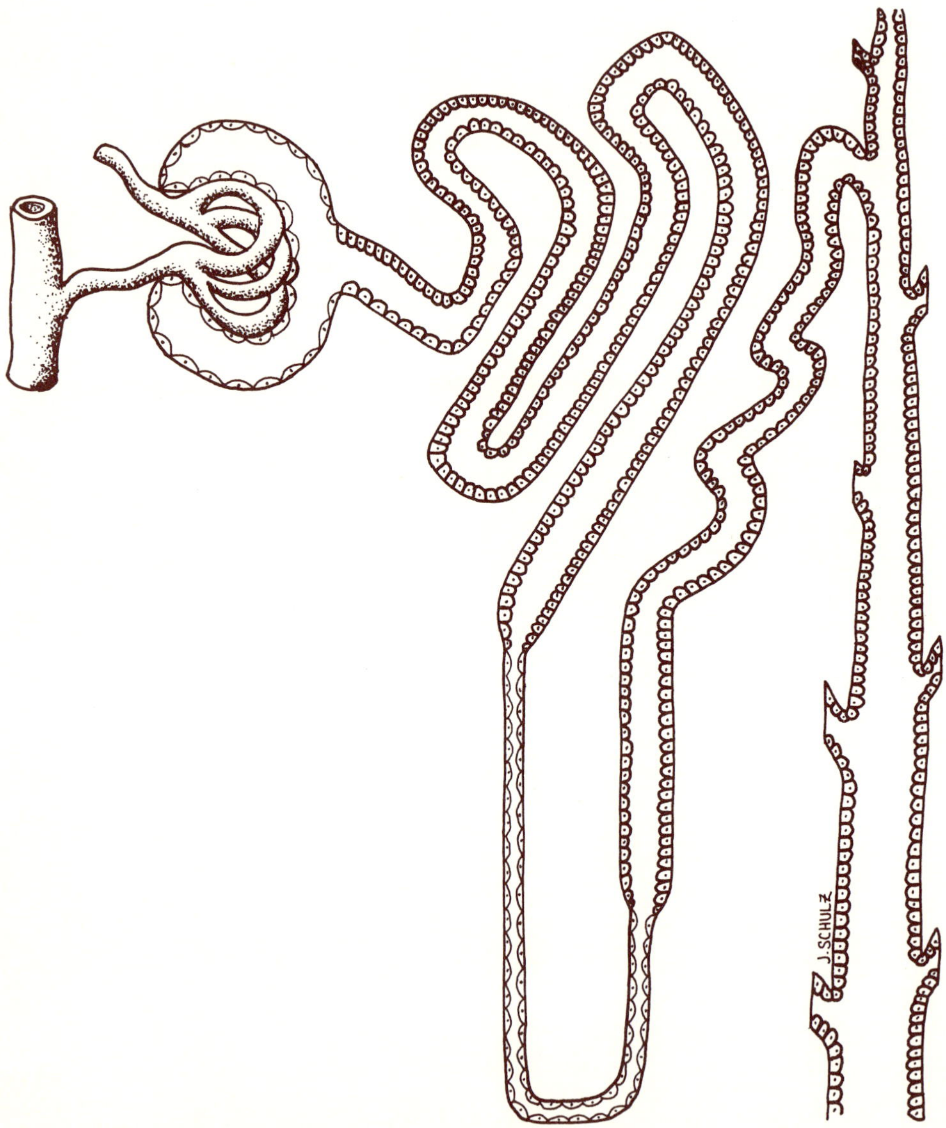

Fig. W-45 Basic structure of a nephron.

Module II: Basic Function of the Nephron and Micturition

Objectives

Upon completion of this module the student will be able to:

1. List the three following basic operations of the nephron (in any order): filtration, secretion, and reabsorption.
2. Define *glomerular filtration* and state the forces that affect it.
3. Identify active and passive processes and the direction of particle movement as examples of secretion or reabsorption according to definitions given in the text.
4. Select the approximate amounts of fluid filtered, reabsorbed, and excreted in the kidney of the human body per day as given in the text.
5. Deduce the three main modes in which substances are handled by filtration, secretion, and reabsorption (see Fig. 11-5, p. 324).
6. Explain how the concept of clearance is used in the measurement of GFR.
7. Describe the relationship between GFR and renal plasma flow.
8. Identify both active and passive processes as parts of tubular reabsorption; explain how one proves that a substance has been reabsorbed.
9. Define *maximal tubular capacity* (T_m).
10. State how plasma composition can be regulated by regulating renal reabsorption and secretion.
11. Given a diagram of the method for measuring glomerular filtration (see Fig. 11-6, p. 326), identify the following: (*a*) a substance suitable for determining GFR, and (*b*) the clearance of a substance as indicated by sample data.
12. Describe tubular secretion; explain how one proves that a substance has been secreted.
13. Differentiate between secretion and excretion.
14. State the muscle actions of the bladder and sphincters during micturition.
15. Describe the neural control of micturition.
16. Contrast the neural control of micturition in an infant with that in an adult.

Reading Assignment

Chap. 11, pp. 323–331.

Supplementary Materials

The following table (p. 124) shows afferent and efferent glomerular arteriolar resistance and effect on filtration pressure.

Afferent Arteriole	Efferent Arteriole	Filtration Pressure
Dilate	——	↑
Dilate	Dilate	↔
Dilate	Constrict	↑↑
Constrict	——	↓
Constrict	Dilate	↓↓
Constrict	Constrict	↔
——	Constrict	↑
——	Dilate	↓
——	——	↔

Renal Plasma Flow

To determine the renal plasma flow, para-aminohippuric acid (PAH) or iodopyracet (Diodrast) are generally infused. They are filtered by the glomeruli and secreted by the tubular cells. The *extraction ratio* is high (arterial concentration minus renal venous concentration/arterial concentration). Since almost all the PAH is completely cleared from the plasma as it flows through the kidney (either by filtration or secretion), the clearance of PAH is a measure of the effective renal plasma flow. The renal plasma flow is calculated by dividing the amount of PAH in the urine by the level of plasma PAH. The PAH concentration of peripheral venous plasma can be used because it is similar to that in the arterial plasma which reaches the kidney. The value obtained is called the *effective renal plasma flow* (ERPF) to indicate that the level in renal venous plasma was not measured. In human beings, the average ERPF values are approximately 625 ml/min.

$$\text{Effective renal plasma flow (ERPF)} = \frac{U_{PAH}V}{P_{PAH}} = \text{clearance of PAH } (C_{PAH})$$

For example:
Concentration of PAH, in urine (U_{PAH}): 14 mg/ml.
Urine volume (V): 0.9 ml/min.
Concentration of PAH in plasma (P_{PAH}): 0.02 mg/ml.

$$\text{ERPF} = \frac{14 \times 0.9}{0.02} = 630 \text{ ml/min}$$

The ERPF determined in this way is the clearance of PAH.

ERPF can also be converted to actual renal plasma flow (RPF). The average PAH extraction ratio is 0.9. (This value is only 90 percent of the total renal plasma flow since about 10 percent of the renal plasma flow supplies nonsecreting portions of the kidneys and therefore cannot lose its PAH by secretion.)

$$\frac{\text{ERPF}}{\text{Extraction ratio}} = \frac{630}{0.9} = \text{actual RPF} = 700 \text{ ml/min}$$

If the hematocrit (Hct) is 45 percent (0.45) then plasma is 55 percent (0.55) and

$$\frac{\text{Renal blood flow}}{\text{Renal plasma flow}} = \frac{1.0}{0.55}$$

and

$$\text{Renal blood flow} = 700 \text{ ml/min} \times \frac{1.0}{0.55} = 1273 \text{ ml/min}$$

Exercises

1. Directions: Write a verbal formula for computing both the GFR and the RPF in the space that follows. (See p. 326 in the text if you need help.)

2. Match the forces given in column A with the pressures (mmHg) given in column B. For whatever pressures you select for the osmotic gradient, hydrostatic pressure, and glomerular capillary blood pressure, calculate the net filtration pressure. (See Table 11-2, p. 325.)

	Column A	Column B (mmHg)
______	Osmotic gradient	*a* 10
______	Hydrostatic pressure in Bowman's capsule	*b* 20
______	Glomerular capillary blood pressure	*c* 30
___X___	Net filtration pressure	*d* 40
		e 50
		f 60

3. Explain the requirements of a material used to measure GFR in terms of filterability, secretion, and reabsorption. *(326)*

4. The percentage of the total plasma which constitutes glomerular filtrate in an average normal person is approximately ______________________________. *(326)*
5. In Fig. W-46 (p. 126), label all the tagged areas and the numbered arrows. Refer to Fig. 11-4, p. 323, to check your answers.
6. The normal micturition process is initiated by receptors in the bladder called ______________________________ receptors. When the signal from these receptors is sufficiently strong a spinal reflex action causes contraction of the smooth muscle in the bladder wall, causing a relaxation of the ______________________________ sphincter. In adults, micturition can be delayed via descending pathways from the cerebral cortex which inhibit ______________________________ nerves to the bladder and stimulate motor nerves to the ______________________________. *(330–331)*

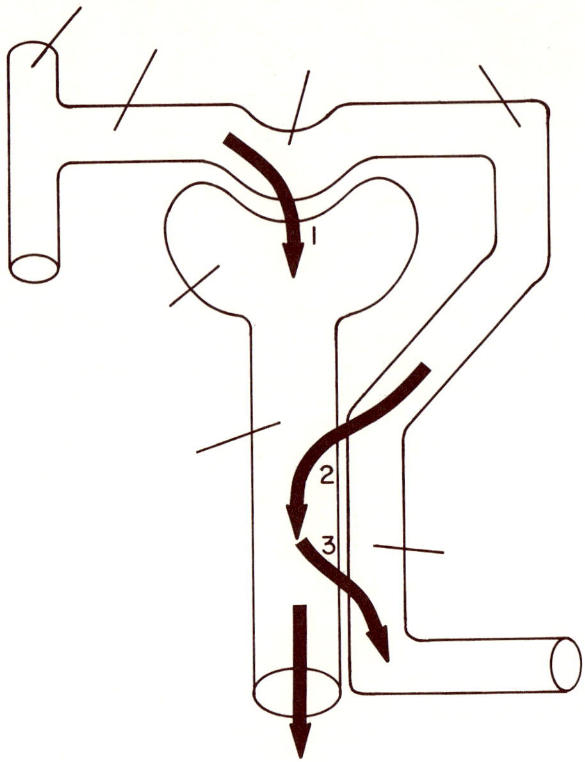

Fig. W-46

Self-Test

Part I

Directions: Circle the correct answer(s).

1. Mrs. Johnson has just had a urinalysis that shows indications of glucose in the urine. The cause(s) for this could be

   a diabetes mellitus.
   b too little glucose in the plasma.
   c the maximal tubular capacity of glucose has been exceeded.
   d faulty reabsorption of glucose.
   e less than double the amount of glucose in the plasma.

2. The amount of fluid filtered from the plasma into Bowman's capsule per day is approximately

   a 220 liters. *b* 140 liters.
   c 180 liters. *d* 100 liters.

3. The average person excretes between ________ and ________ of urine per day.

   a 160–180 liters   *b* 1–3 mg
   c 1–2 ml   *d* 1–2 liters

4. If Mr. Collins's kidney filters the average amount of fluid per day, approximately what fraction of this fluid would be reabsorbed into the peritubular capillaries per day?

   a 99 percent   *b* 10 percent   *c* 50 percent   *d* 1 percent

Part II

Directions: Figs. W-47 through W-50 are simple diagrams of the four main modes of renal manipulation of substances. Briefly describe the mode depicted by each diagram. Substance A has been given as an example.

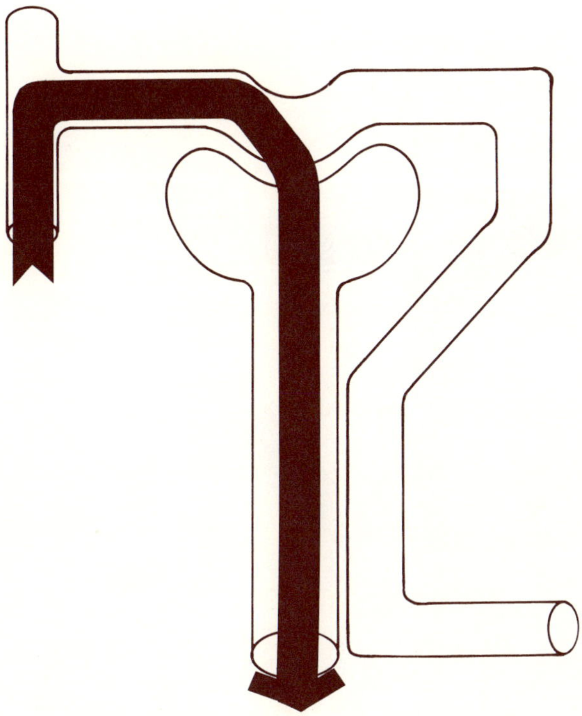

Fig. W-47 Substance A is handled by filtration only.

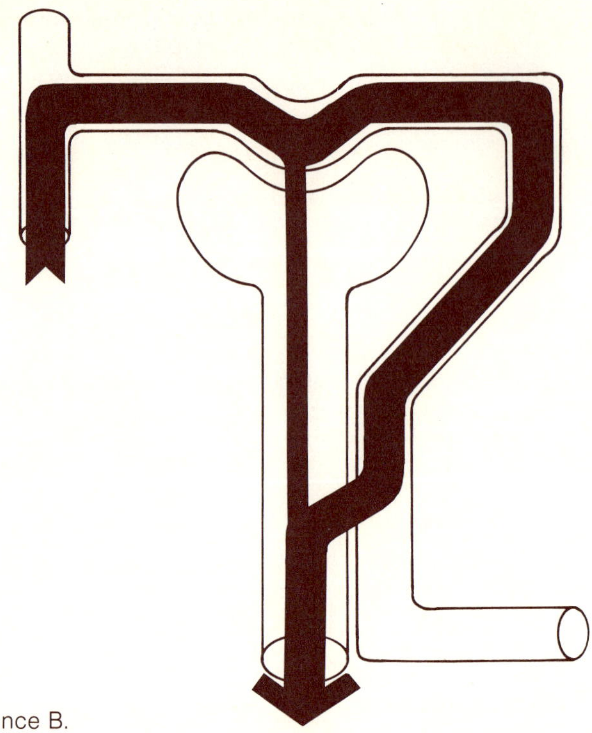

Fig. W-48 Substance B.

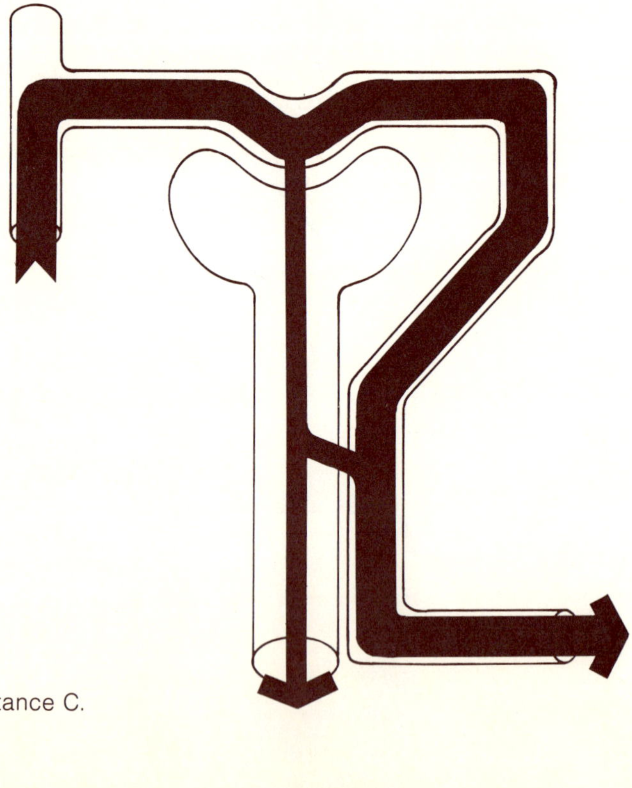

Fig. W-49 Substance C.

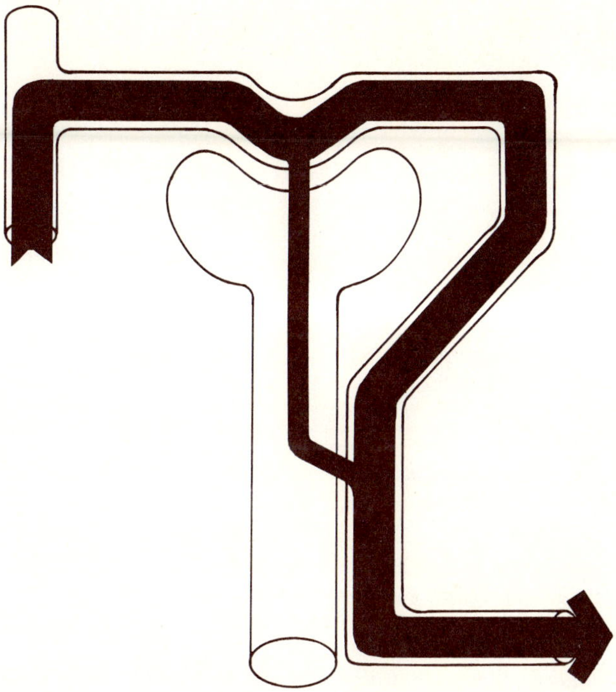

Fig. W-50 Substance D.

Part III

Directions: Answer the following questions in the space provided.

1. Briefly describe the characteristics of the substance used to determine GFR and give an example of such a substance.

   Characteristics: ____________________

   ____

   Example: ____________________

   ____

2. Provided below are the data collected. Compute GFR.

Volume of urine collected during 24-hr period	2 liters/day
Amount of filtered substance (*W*) in urine	700 mg
Plasma W concentration	3.5 mg/liter

   GFR =

3. Assuming the glomerular filtrate constitutes one-fifth the total plasma entering the kidney, compute the renal plasma flow (RPF).

   RPF =

4. If the concentration of protein in the glomerular filtrate was 0.005 g per 100 ml and none was reabsorbed, how much protein would be excreted per day assuming a normal GFR of about 180 l/day?* ____________________
5. The hospital lab reports that your patient's creatinine clearance is 120 g/day. This value is:

   a normal *b* significantly below normal
   c nonsense
6. The following test results were obtained on specimens from a person over a 24-hr period. Total urine volume = 1.4 liters.

   U_{In} = 100 mg/100 ml U_{PAH} = 700 mg/ml
   P_{In} = 1 mg/100 ml P_{PAH} = 2 mg/ml
   U_{urea} = 220 m*M*/liter P_{urea} = 5 m*M*/liter

   a What are the clearances of inulin? ____________________

   Urea? ____________________

   PAH? ____________________

   b How much urea is reabsorbed? ____________________
   c How much PAH is secreted (assuming no PAH reabsorption and complete filtration of PAH)? ____________________
7. An increase in the plasma concentration of inulin causes (an increase, a decrease, no change) in the renal clearance of inulin. ____________________
8. The clearance of substance A is less than that simultaneously determined for inulin. Give three possible explanations.

   a ____________________

   b ____________________

   c ____________________
9. If 50 percent of the nephrons were destroyed, which of the following compounds would be likely to show an increased blood concentration?

   a urea *b* most amino acids
   c glucose *d* purines

* Questions 4 to 9 reprinted from Vander, *Renal Physiology*, McGraw-Hill, New York, 1975.

Module III: Regulation of the Renal Function, Part I

Objectives

Upon completion of this module the student will be able to

1. Summarize the tubular mechanisms for handling sodium, chloride, and water by the kidney.
2. Describe antidiuretic hormone and its role in the kidney.
3. State the two determinants of sodium excretion rate.
4. State the three factors that determine glomerular filtration rates.
5. Describe the reflex pathway by which GFR is regulated (see Fig. 11-14, p. 335).
6. Describe the reflex pathway by which tubular sodium reabsorption is regulated (see Fig. 11-16, p. 337).
7. Describe the relation between renin, angiotensin, and aldosterone (see Fig. 11-15, p. 336).
8. Define *third factor.*
9. Describe the reflex pathway by which water excretion is altered in response to changes in extracellular volume (see Figs. 11-17, 11-18, p. 338).
10. Describe the reflex pathway by which water excretion is altered in response to changes in plasma osmolarity (see Fig. 11-21, p. 342).
11. Describe how the countercurrent system produces a hyperosmotic interstitium in the renal medulla; state how either a hypotonic or hypertonic urine is formed.
12. Describe the stimuli which promote thirst.
13. Describe the role of the hypothalamic centers in mediating thirst.
14. Describe salt appetite.

Reading Assignment

Chap. 11, pp. 331–345.

Exercises

Part I

Directions: In each of the following items, fill in the blank following each phrase to indicate the change in direction of excretion of Na, Cl, and H_2O under the conditions described. The first part of question 1 is given as an example. Figure 11-12 in the text will be particularly helpful in completing this exercise.

1. When the GFR is normal and reabsorption of Na increases

   a Na excretion decreases ______.

   b Cl excretion ______.

   c H_2O excretion ______.

2. When the GFR increases and Na reabsorption remains the same

   a Na excretion ______.

   b Cl excretion ______.

   c H_2O excretion ______.

3. When GFR increases and Na reabsorption decreases

   a Na excretion ______.

   b Cl excretion ______.

   c H_2O excretion ______.

4. When GFR is normal and Na reabsorption decreases

   a Na excretion ______.

   b Cl excretion ______.

   c H_2O excretion ______.

5. Following salt and water loss due to diarrhea, indicate the direction of change in the following variables (increase ↑ or decrease ↓): *(335–338)*

   a plasma volume
   b GFR
   c filtered Na
   d plasma ADH
   e collecting duct permeability
   f urine volume
   g aldosterone secretion
   h renin secretion
   i cardiac output
   j Na excreted
   k tubular Na reabsorption

6. Show increase or decrease by completing the arrow to the left of each substance. (Refer to Fig. 11-16, p. 337, to check your answers.)

   ↓ plasma volume
   ↓
   | activity of renal sympathetic nerves
   ↓
   | renin secretion
   ↓
   | plasma angiotensin
   ↓
   | aldosterone secretion
   ↓
   | plasma aldosterone
   ↓
   | tubular Na reabsorption
   ↓
   | Na excretion

7. It appears that a third factor as yet unknown is involved in control of renal reabsorption because of what conditions occasionally existing in a person? *(336)*

8. The type of receptors which control ADH secretion by sensing plasma volume is known as ______________________. (337)
9. Active sodium transport does *not* occur in which segment of the loop of Henle?

______________________ (339)

10. Diagram Henle's loop and an associated collecting duct. Assuming a normal plasma sodium concentration of 300 mosm, and a maximum sodium concentration of 1400 mosm, write in the concentration gradients existing and the direction of sodium and water movements. See Fig. 11-20, p. 342, to check your answers.

11. The hypothalamic area responsible for ADH secretion receives neural input from two types of sensory cells called ______________________ and

______________________. (342)

Self-Test

Part I

Directions: Complete Chart 1 using an "I" to indicate an increase in excretion rate, a "D" to indicate a decrease in excretion rate, and an "N" to indicate no change in excretion rate. The GFR and Na reabsorption rates are given. ADH is present and constant.

Chart 1

GFR	Na Reabsorption	Na Excretion	Cl Excretion	H_2O Excretion
N	D			
N	I			
I	D			
I	I			

Part II

Directions: Circle the correct answer(s).

1. Complete inhibition of active sodium reabsorption would cause an increase in the excretion of which of the following substances?

   a water *b* urea
   c chloride *d* glucose

2. Which of the following are true of antidiuretic hormone (ADH)?

   a It increases the water permeability of the collecting ducts and the distal tubules.
   b When large amounts are present, the urine excreted has a high osmolarity.
   c Its absence would cause dehydration through large volumes of urine being excreted.
   d It enables proper functioning of the countercurrent multiplier system because it has no direct effect on sodium reabsorption, only on water reabsorption.

3. Which of the following factors directly affect GFR?

   a plasma sodium concentration
   b plasma calcium concentration
   c glomerular capillary blood pressure
   d Bowman's capsule hydrostatic pressure
   e osmotic pressure due to plasma protein concentration

4. Which of the following correctly describe the reflex pathway relating extracellular volume and water excretion?

   a ADH is produced by a group of hypothalamic neurons whose axons terminate in the posterior pituitary, from which ADH is released into the blood.
   b Vascular baroreceptors particularly in the left atrium send information to the hypothalamic neurons related to ADH secretion.
   c The atrial baroreceptors are stimulated by increased atrial blood pressure and in turn send impulses via ascending pathways to the hypothalamus to stimulate ADH producing cells.
   d Decreased atrial pressure causes less firing by the baroreceptors and more inhibition of ADH synthesis and release.

5. Which of the following are stimuli which promote thirst?

   a drinking ocean salt water
   b lower extracellular volume
   c higher extracellular volume
   d higher plasma osmolarity
   e dryness of throat and mouth

6. Which of the following accurately describe the countercurrent system operation in the kidney?

   a Active sodium chloride transport occurs in the descending limb of the loop of Henle.
   b The countercurrent system could not operate very long without active sodium chloride transport.
   c The highest concentration of sodium chloride is at the tip of the loop of Henle.
   d The final urine sodium chloride concentration can never be greater than that at the tip of the loop of Henle.
   e If no water is lost in the collecting ducts, the urine will be hypertonic.
   f The fluid in the descending limb of Henle is always hypoosmotic relative to that of the ascending limb.
   g The real function of the loop countercurrent multiplier system is to concentrate the medullary interstitium.
   h Maximum sodium chloride concentration is a function of the length of the loop of Henle and the strength of the sodium pump.
   i No ADH control also means no control of sodium chloride concentration in the urine.

j Final urine concentration occurs in the collecting ducts.
k Hypertonic urine results from low levels of ADH.
l Hypertonic urine is possible because ADH allows water to pass out of the collecting tubules until equilibrium with the medullary interstitium is attained.

Module IV: Regulation of the Renal Function, Part II

Objectives

Upon completion of this module, the student will be able to

1. Identify renal control mechanisms and hormonal control of K^+ (Figs. 11-23 and 11-24, pp. 345–346).
2. Identify the mechanisms controlling extracellular calcium concentration by identifying the controlling hormones and the glands from which they originate, and the substance stimulating hormone secretion.
3. Describe the role vitamin D plays in calcium metabolism.
4. Define *acid, base,* and *acidity.*
5. Contrast strong with weak acids.
6. Describe buffering.
7. List the three major sources of hydrogen ion within the body.
8. State the roles of the kidneys and lungs in hydrogen ion excretion.
9. State the roles of bicarbonate and hemoglobin as buffers.
10. State the mechanisms of hydrogen ion excretion by the kidney.
11. State the role of NH_3 and HPO_4 urinary buffers.
12. Define *pyelonephritis* and *glomerulonephritis.*
13. List the symptoms that one would expect in patients with advanced renal disease.
14. Describe the artificial kidney.

Reading Assignment

Pp. 345–354.

Supplementary Materials

You should be able to describe respiratory and metabolic acidosis and alkalosis in terms of the defect, cause, and compensation (see Table 1, p. 136).

Table 1

Condition	Defect				Cause	Compensation
	pH	$[H^+]$	$PaCO_2$	$[HCO_3]$		
Metabolic acidosis	↓	↑	—	↓ *	Renal failure Diarrhea Hypoxia, lactic acid Ketones (diabetes mellitus)	Respiratory alkalosis—hyperventilation resulting in ↓ $PaCO_2$ (also renal compensations)
Metabolic alkalosis	↑	↓	—	↑ *	Vomiting $NaHCO_3$ ingestion Infusion of HCO_3^- Diuretics	Respiratory acidosis—hypoventilation resulting in ↑ $PaCO_2$ (also renal compensations)
Respiratory alkalosis	↑	↓	↓ *	↓ (slight)	Hyperventilation Anesthesia (hyperventilation) Neurotic hyperventilation	Metabolic acidosis—HCO_3^- depletion by kidney Increased lactic acid formation Decreased H^+ secretion by kidney
Respiratory acidosis	↓	↑	↑ *	↑ (slight)	Decreased pulmonary function Decreased cardiac output Sedation resulting in decreased respiratory drive Neuromuscular blockade Chronic obstructive disease	Metabolic alkalosis—increased kidney reabsorption of HCO_3^- Increased H^+ secretion by kidney

* Primary defect.

Exercises

Directions: Answer each question below in the space provided.

1. Identify the site and basic regulatory process of H^+ ion regulation in the kidney. *(353)*

Site: ____________________

Basic regulatory process: ____________________

2. Identify the two major hydrogen ion buffers found in the urine. *(353)*

 a ____________________ *b* ____________________

3. Briefly note what occurs in hydrogen ion regulation in the kidney under the following circumstances (pp. 353–354 in the text will be helpful in completing this exercise).

 a Absence of buffers in the urine ____________________

 ____

 b Occurrence of a high concentration of hydrogen ions in the urine in the presence of NH_3 ____________________

 ____

 c Persistence of a high concentration of hydrogen ions in the extracellular fluid for one to two days ____________________

 ____

4. Write a formula describing the HPO_4^- buffering action on the hydrogen ion. *(353)*

5. Complete the arrows to show an increase or a decrease in the components of the pathway shown. (See Fig. 11-25, page 347, to check your answers.)

↓↑ plasma volume

↓

| renin secretion

↓

| plasma renin

↓

| plasma angiotensin | plasma potassium

| aldosterone secretion

↓

| plasma aldosterone

| tubular secretion of potassium | tubular reabsorption of sodium

↓ ↓

| potassium excretion | sodium excretion

6. What are the two most important factors controlling potassium levels? ______________

____ (346)

7. Which is more important in controlling potassium levels, filtration, reabsorption, or secretion? ______________________________ (345)

8. (a) Name two hormones which are important in controlling plasma calcium levels. (b) What glands secrete these hormones? (c) What substance controls their secretion? (347–349)

   a ____

   b ____

   c ____

9. Explain the difference between the items in each of the following pairs and give examples of each. (349–350)

   a acid-base

   b strong-acid–weak-acid

   c buffer-acidity

10. How do the lungs participate in acid-base balance? (351)

11. Two very important buffers in the human body are bicarbonate and hemoglobin. Write equations for each of these showing how they act as buffers in the body. (351, 353)

12. How does the kidney excrete hydrogen ions utilizing the two major urinary buffers HPO_4^- and NH_3? (353–354)

13. Describe the symptoms of advanced glomerulonephritis. (354)

14. How does the artificial kidney work? (354)

Self-Test

Part I

Directions: Circle the correct answer(s).

1. In hydrogen ion regulation in the kidney

   a reabsorption is the primary regulatory mechanism.
   b secretion is the primary regulatory mechanism.
   c both secretion and reabsorption are regulatory processes.
   d the site of regulation is Bowman's capsule.
   e the site of regulation occurs between the tubular lumen and peritubular capillaries.
   f the site of regulation is the urethra.

2. During hydrogen ion buffering in the kidney

   a NH_3 combines with H^+ to become NH_4^+.
   b HPO_4^{2-} combines with H^+ to become $H_2PO_4^-$.
   c decreased hydrogen ion concentration results in increased NH_3 excretion in the form of NH_4^+.
   d the amount of ammonia which remains in the tubular lumen depends upon the rate of hydrogen ion secretion.

Part II

Directions: Complete the following items in the space provided.

1. Both parathormone and calcitonin secretions are controlled directly by

   ______________________________.

2. The three major sources of hydrogen ion in the body are ______________________________

   ____.

Part III

Directions: Circle T for true and F for false.

T F 1. Two important factors in renal regulation of potassium are aldosterone levels and potassium concentration of the renal tubular cell.

T F 2. Aldosterone has the same effect on potassium as it does on sodium in renal control since they are similar chemically.

T F 3. Calcium levels in the bloodstream are controlled by parathormone and ADH.

T F 4. Parathormone production is controlled via the hypothalamic-pituitary tracts and neural reflex control similar to sodium.

T F 5. Parathormone and calcitonin control are opposing systems for potassium regulation.

T F 6. The major action of vitamin D is to stimulate active calcium absorption by the intestine.

T F 7. The lungs and the kidneys are the only normal sources of hydrogen ion elimination in the body.

T F 8. The lungs function to remove hydrogen ion from plasma by providing for the elimination of carbon dioxide via the reaction $H^+ + HCO_3^- \rightarrow H_2CO_3 \rightarrow CO_2 + H_2O$.

T F 9. The primary control of hydrogen ion excretion in the kidney is the direct effect of hydrogen ion concentration on the tubular cells.

T F 10. In general, the kidney controls hydrogen ion excretion by filtration, reabsorption, and secretion.

T F 11. Hemoglobin functions to buffer hydrogen ions while they are in transit from the tissues to the lungs.

Part IV

Directions: Match the items in column A with those in column B. Each item may be used more than once. Also, there may be more than one match.

	Column A	Column B
1. ______	Substance which can accept a hydrogen ion.	*a* base
2. ______	Degree of hydrogen ion concentration.	*b* acid
3. ______	Compound capable of liberating a hydrogen ion.	*c* acidity
4. ______	Dissociates completely when dissolved in water.	*d* strong acid
5. ______	Only partially dissociates when dissolved in water.	*e* weak acid
6. ______	HCl is an example.	*f* buffer
7. ______	H_2CO_3 is an example.	*g* buffering
8. ______	Lactic acid is an example.	*h* hormone
9. ______	Process of preventing large changes in hydrogen ion contration when hydrogen ions are added or removed from a solution.	
10. ______	Hemoglobin is an example.	

Part V

Directions: Circle the correct answer(s).

1. Which of the following are true of renal regulation of potassium?

   a Like sodium, potassium is completely filterable at the glomerulus.
   b Potassium can be reabsorbed but not secreted by the tubules.
   c Potassium is not filterable at the glomerulus, but is secreted by the renal tubules.
   d Reabsorption is not a controlling factor of potassium homeostasis.
   e Potassium excretory changes are primarily due to changes in secretion.
   f Normal GFR changes do not measurably alter the control of potassium secretion.
   g The hormone aldosterone reduces tubular potassium secretion.
   h An important control factor is tubule cellular potassium concentration via a concentration gradient with the lumen and passive moment to or from it.

2. High calcium levels in the extracellular plasma promote which of the following?

   a increased parathormone secretion
   b decreased parathormone secretion

c increased ADH secretion
d decreased ADH secretion
e increased calcitonin secretion
f decreased calcitonin secretion

3. Which are major sources of hydrogen ion in the body?

a bile salts
b hormones
c inorganic acids such as phosphoric and sulfuric acids
d carbonic acid
e organic acids from metabolic reactions

4. Which of the following describe the buffer role of bicarbonate in the equation

$$H^+ + HCO_3^- \underset{2}{\overset{1}{\rightleftharpoons}} H_2CO_3 \underset{4}{\overset{3}{\rightleftharpoons}} H_2O + CO_2$$

a Increased hydrogen ion prompts reaction 1.
b Decreased hydrogen ion prompts reactions 2 and 4.
c All four reactions occur simultaneously in the body.
d Reaction 3 occurs mostly in body tissues.

CHAPTER 12

DIGESTION AND ABSORPTION OF FOOD

Module I:
Structure and Regulation of the GI System; Physiology of Salivation and Swallowing

Module II:
Stomach

Module III:
Pancreatic Secretions; Secretion of Bile

Module IV:
Small and Large Intestine

Module I: Structure and Regulation of the GI System; Physiology of Salivation and Swallowing

Objectives

Upon completion of this module the student will be able to:

1. Label a diagram of the anatomy of the gastrointestinal tract with the following items: parotid salivary gland, pharynx, trachea, esophagus, sublingual and submaxillary (submandibular) salivary glands, diaphragm, stomach, pancreas, small intestine, large intestine, gallbladder, liver, appendix, rectum, and anus.
2. Draw a simple line diagram of a segment of the small intestine and label the following structures: serosa, three muscle layers—longitudinal smooth, circular smooth, muscularis mucosae; submucosa; mucosa; and nerve plexuses.
3. List the three efferent pathways that influence the activity of intestinal smooth muscle and exocrine glands.
4. List at least four stimuli perceived by the central nervous system (afferent inputs) that are capable of initiating the efferent pathways in objective 3 above.
5. List the four intraluminal stimuli that initiate the efferent pathways in objective 3 above.
6. List the three pairs of exocrine glands which produce saliva.
7. List the three major components of saliva.
8. List the stimuli for initiation of salivation.
9. Explain the fact that swallowing is both voluntary and reflex.
10. Describe the act of swallowing.
11. State the function of the gastroesophageal sphincter.
12. State the physiological reasons for "heartburn" during the last five months of pregnancy.

Reading Assignment

Chap. 12, pp. 355–363.

Exercises

The F.B.I. (Fats, Bile, Intestinal) Story—Part I

At 5:02 P.M. on Saturday, August 8, the subject George Peabody (also known as G. I. George) was seen loitering outside Mama's Little Pizza Parlor on the east side. Positive

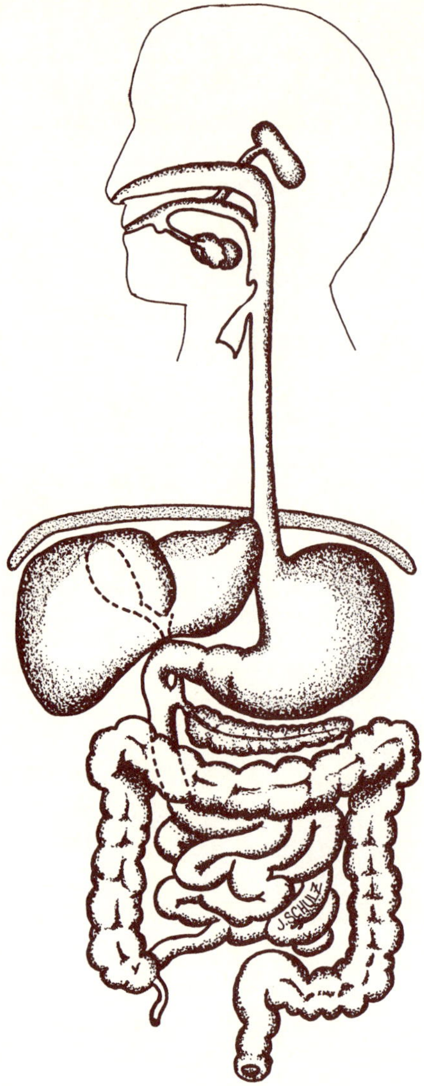

Fig. W-51 Anatomy of the GI tract.

identification of the subject was made using the composite diagrams of his GI tract as shown in Fig. W-51.

Label Fig. W-51 with the following clues: parotid salivary gland, pharynx, trachea, esophagus, sublingual and submaxillary salivary glands, diaphragm, stomach, pancreas, small intestine, large intestine, gallbladder, liver, appendix, rectum, anus. (See Fig. 12-1, p. 356, for help.)

Label Fig. W-52 with the following: three muscle layers, submucosal layer, mucosal layer nerve plexuses. (See Fig. 12-3, p. 358, to check your answers.)

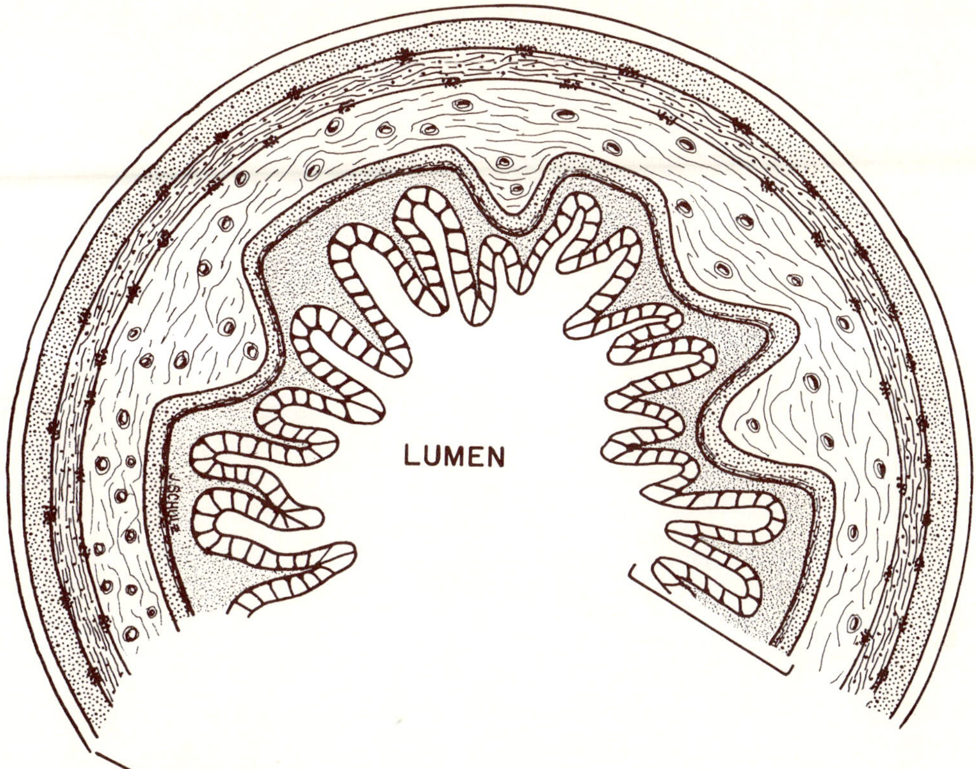

Fig. W-52 Anatomy of the small intestine.

At 5:04 P.M. G. I. George was still waiting for his contact to appear when certain stimuli perceived by his central nervous system activated the three efferent pathways that influence the activity of intestinal smooth muscle and exocrine glands. Name four stimuli emanating from a carry-out order of pizza with double anchovies that are capable of initiating GI reflexes.

a ______________________________

b ______________________________

c ______________________________

d ______________________________ (*360, Fig. 12-5*)

The three efferent pathways stimulated were:

a ______________________________

b ______________________________

c ______________________________ (*358*)

At 5:05 P.M. George's contact still had not shown. He decided to wait inside Mama's Parlor, and, just for something to do, provide a major stimulation for salivation. What was George going to do? ____

____ (*361*)

That's right. George ordered his favorite pizza with the "works" (also known as the "Heartburn Special"). While contemplating the events of the night to come (and his pizza), George's mouth began to water. The following three exocrine glands were identified as those suspected of producing the saliva.

Exhibit A: ____

Exhibit B: ____

Exhibit C: ____ (*359*)

It is believed that a sample of saliva taken at this time would have revealed the following major components:

a ____________________ *b* ____________________ (*359–360*)

c ____________________

After the pizza arrived, George gobbled down the first bite upon which nestled an anchovy. George loved this little morsel, but his gastroesophageal sphincter had some difficulty deciding whether to accept it or not. What function does the gastroesophageal normally serve? ____

____ (*362*)

Still keeping an eye out for his contact, George gulped down the pizza without any problems in 12 minutes flat. At 5:28 P.M. he saw her—a dame holding one kid by the hand, and with another on the way. He was sure this was the contact he had been waiting for. He returned to the corner where he had been standing and waited for the woman to approach him with the passwords. It was her, all right. She said, "I've got heartburn." George's countersign phrase is a physiological explanation for why a woman who is over five months pregnant has heartburn (assuming she has not just eaten a Heartburn Special). What does George say to his contact? (*363*)

Tune in to Module II for the next episode of the F.B.I. story.

Self-Test

Part I

Directions: On Fig. W-53, a diagram of the anatomy of the gastrointestinal tract, label the following items:

a parotid salivary gland
b pharynx
c trachea
d esophagus
e sublingual and submaxillary salivary glands
f diaphragm
g stomach
h pancreas
i small intestine
j large intestine
k gallbladder
l liver
m appendix
n rectum
o anus

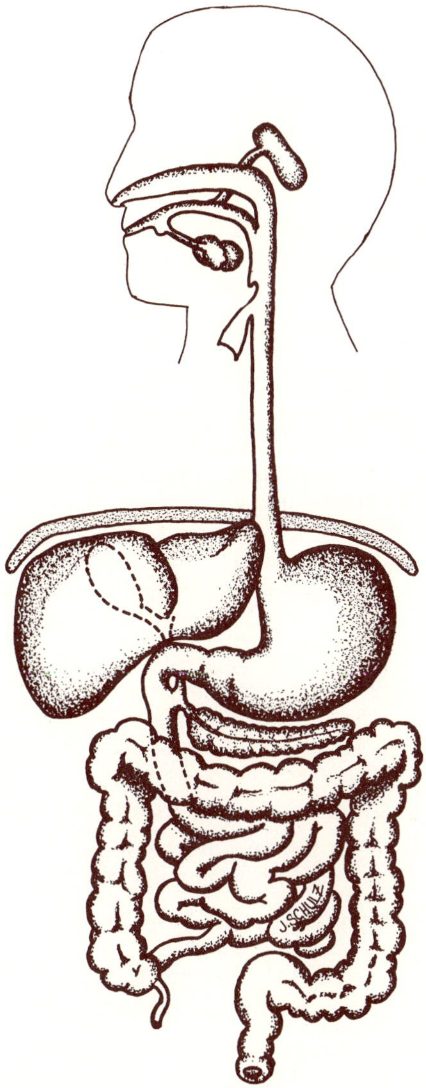

Fig. W-53

Part II

Directions: In the space provided below, draw a simple diagram of a segment of the small intestine and label the following structures:

a serosa
b three muscle layers: longitudinal smooth, circular smooth, muscularis mucosae
c mucosa
d submucosa
e nerve plexuses

Part III

Directions: Answer the following questions in the space provided.

1. List the three efferent pathways that influence the activity of intestinal smooth muscle and exocrine glands.

   a ______ *b* ______ *c* ______

2. List the three pairs of major exocrine glands which produce saliva.

   a ______ *b* ______ *c* ______

3. List at least three of the four intraluminal stimuli that initiate the efferent pathways that influence the activity of intestinal smooth muscle and exocrine glands.

   a ______ *b* ______

   c ______ *d* ______

Part IV

Directions: Circle the correct answer(s).

1. John has just passed by a pastry shop filled with mouth-watering goodies. If John's mouth does, in fact, "water," which of the following statements are true?

   a The stimuli of sight triggered a reaction in the central nervous system.
   b Proteins, salts, and water formed the "watery secretions."
   c Hormones secreted by the pituitary gland helped to stimulate salivation.
   d The sublingual gland, submaxillary gland, and parotid gland's secretions combined to form saliva.

2. Sally just had the agonizing experience of having a piece of food "go down the wrong way." What happened?

a The gastroesophageal sphincter failed to relax.
b The piece of food entered the trachea.
c The glottis did not close.
d The hypopharyngeal sphincter did not close.

3. The gastroesophageal sphincter

a is relaxed when swallowing is *not* taking place.
b provides a barrier between the diaphragm and the stomach.
c is relaxed when a peristaltic wave begins in the esophagus.
d prevents internal pressure in the stomach from pushing food into the esophagus.
e may cause achalasia when it fails to function correctly.

4. During the last five months of pregnancy, "heartburn"

a may occur because of decreased pressure in the abdominal cavity.
b symptoms may disappear in the last weeks of pregnancy.
c tends to occur because the gastroesophageal sphincter becomes constricted.
d seldom occurs.

Part V

Directions: Circle T for true and F for false.

T F 1. The human being must thoroughly chew food before swallowing to assure adequate digestion.
T F 2. Emotions may stimulate efferent pathways that influence the intestinal smooth muscle.
T F 3. Stimulation of chemoreceptors and pressure receptors in the mouth initiates salivation.
T F 4. Digestive activity begins in the stomach.
T F 5. Nerves alone control the secretion of saliva.
T F 6. Chewing on a marble would tend to initiate salivation even though there is no food in the mouth.
T F 7. Most of the saliva secreted is swallowed without reacting with food.
T F 8. The most potent stimuli for salivation are alkaline solutions, such as milk.
T F 9. The newborn child tends to regurgitate because the glottis is not fully developed.

Module II: **Stomach**

Objectives

Upon completion of this module the student will be able to:

1. Label the following items on a diagram of the anatomy of the stomach: esophagus, fundus, body, antrum, pyloric sphincter, and duodenum.

2. Identify the characteristics of the chyme and the basic electrical rhythm.
3. List the factors influencing the rate of gastric emptying.
4. Describe secretin and cholecystokinin, their chemical nature, site of origin, and stimulus for release.
5. List the three efferent pathways controlling gastric motility.
6. Describe the process of vomiting by listing the sequence of steps that occur during vomiting.
7. List the three functions of HCl secretion in the stomach.
8. State the locations of both HCl and pepsin secretion.
9. Identify the function of the enzyme pepsin.
10. Identify the characteristics of the cephalic, gastric, and intestinal phase of gastric secretion.
11. List at least four factors in the duodenum that influence gastric secretion.
12. Identify the function, site of production, and stimuli causing release of gastrin.
13. Identify two efferent pathways (other than gastric hormones) which lead to an increase in acid and enzyme secretion in the stomach.
14. List the factors that increase acid and enzyme secretion in the stomach (see Fig. 12-15, p. 371).
15. List two effects secretin and CCK have on the stomach.
16. Describe GI ulceration; state the sites of its most frequent occurrences (see pages 371–372).

Reading Assignment

Chap. 12, pp. 363–373. Prepare yourself for a slightly longer than average module.

Supplementary Materials

Postprandial alkalosis:
From Fig. 12-19, p. 375, it is clear that as H^+ ions are secreted into the lumen of the stomach, HCO_3^- ions are added to the blood, leading to a raised pH. This has been called postprandial alkalosis.

Definitions:

Enterogastrones: Since secretin and CCK are produced in the duodenum and their site of action is the stomach, they are often referred to as the enterogastrones.
Pancreozymin: This is an alternate name for cholecystokinin (see p. 376).

Exercises

Part I

Directions: Fill in the blanks in the following sentences with the missing words. See pp. 366–367 for help.

Hal has just finished his last final exam and he and some of the guys in the class decide to celebrate in one of the local eateries. They consume a huge amount of pizza and an unbelievable amount (well, a lot, anyway) of beer. All of a sudden, four things happen to Hal that generally precede vomiting. What are they? *(366)*

a ______________________________

b ______________________________

c ______________________________

d ______________________________

It becomes apparent to Hal that his vomiting center has received a message from his stomach regarding impending vomiting. Where is the vomiting center located?

______________________________ *(367)*

Just as Hal reaches the nearest men's room, the process of vomiting begins with the following occurrences: *(366)*

a ______________________________

b ______________________________

c ______________________________

Soon after, Hal's thoracic and abdominal muscles contract causing a rise in pressure in the ______________________________. This increase in pressure causes *(366)* relaxation of the ______________________________ (two words). The pizza and beer are pushed into the esophagus as the result of *(366)*

a ______________________________

b ______________________________

Hal returns to the table to assure his friends that he is feeling much better.

Part II

The F.B.I. Story—Part II

At 5:30 P.M. on Saturday, August 8, G. I. George confirms that the woman outside Mama's Little Pizza Parlor is his contact, known to him only by the name of Hilda. He reaches into his coat pocket for the microfilm he is to transfer to Hilda. It's gone! He had noticed a small crunchy piece of something on his pizza that he thought was probably just an anchovy bone, but it must have been the microfilm. By now it is churning around in his stomach with the Heartburn Special. George suggests a quick trip to the local medical school for help in retrieving the film.

At the emergency room of the school medical center, G. I. George explains his predicament to the attending intern (luckily, someone who is sympathetic to his cause).

The physician explains that the microfilm may already be an integral part of the chyme. George wants to know what chyme is. Tell him. ______________________________

______________________________ *(363)*

The physician also explains about the basic electrical rhythm of the stomach and its relation to stomach motility. What does he say? *(364)*

Since he is unable to x-ray George (an x-ray would ruin the film), the doctor attempts to trace the film using logical methods. He begins by looking in a physiology text to find the factors influencing gastric emptying. Fill him in on the stomach and its activities by answering the questions below.

1. List the factors influencing gastric emptying. *(365)*

2. List the three functions of HCl secretion in the stomach.

   a ____________________

   b ____________________

   c ____________________ *(367)*

3. Identify the locations of HCl and pepsin secretion.

   HCl: ____________________

   Pepsin: ____________________ *(367)*

4. Describe the function of the enzyme pepsin. ____________________

   ____________________ *(368)*

5. Identify the characteristics of the cephalic phase of gastric secretion. ____________________

   ____________________ *(369)*

6. List four factors in the duodenum that influence gastric secretion.

   a ____________________

   b ____________________

   c ____________________

   d ____________________ *(370)*

7. Identify the function, site of production, and stimuli causing release of gastrin.

   Function: ____________________

   Site of production: ____________________

   Stimuli: ____________________ *(369–370)*

8. List two factors other than gastric hormones which lead to an increase in acid and enzyme secretion in the stomach.

   a ____________________

   b ____________________ *(370–371)*

9. List two effects secretin and CCK have on the stomach.

   a ____________________

   b ____________________ *(365)*

10. Identify two sites of frequent ulceration.

   a ______________________________

   b ______________________________ (*371*)

With these facts in hand, the physician decides it's too late to operate and that all G. I. George can do is sit and wait it out. Follow the progress of G. I. George in the next module.

Self-Test

Part I

Directions: On the diagram of the anatomy of the stomach provided in Fig. W-55, label the following items:

a esophagus *b* fundus *c* body
d antrum *e* pyloric sphincter *f* duodenum

Part II

Directions: Answer each question below in the space provided.

1. What is chyme? ______________________________

2. List the three efferent pathways controlling gastric motility.

   a ______________________________

   b ______________________________

   c ______________________________

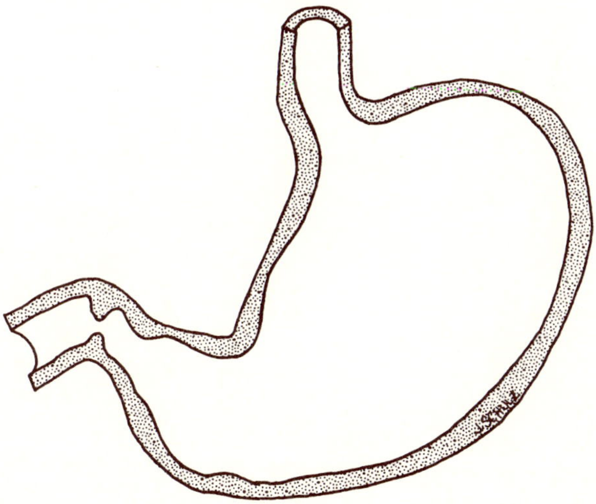

Fig. W-55

3. List the three functions of HCl secretion in the stomach.

   a ______________________________

   b ______________________________

   c ______________________________

4. List four factors in the duodenum that influence gastric secretion.

   a ______________________________

   b ______________________________

   c ______________________________

   d ______________________________

5. List two sites of frequent ulceration.

   a ______________________________

   b ______________________________

6. List the three general pathways which control acid and enzyme secretion in the stomach.

   a ______________________________

   b ______________________________

   c ______________________________

Part III

Directions: Circle the correct answer(s).

1. Gastric emptying

   a is aided by relaxation of muscles at the antrum.
   b increases when the presence of acid in the duodenum is elevated.
   c begins when weak peristaltic waves move over the body of the stomach.
   d is the process whereby chyme gets moved from the stomach into the large intestine.

2. Secretin and cholecystokinin (CCK)

   a are hormones.
   b originate in the body of the stomach.
   c are secreted in response to the presence of amino acids or fatty acids in the lumen of the duodenum.
   d decrease the rate of gastric secretion and emptying.

3. Vomiting may be caused by

   a tactile stimulation in the back of the throat.
   b intense pain.
   c ingestion of certain chemical agents.
   d increased pressure within the skull.

4. HCl

   a secretion inhibits enzyme release in the stomach.
   b kills most of the bacteria entering the stomach with food.

c continues the process of reducing large particles of food to smaller particles in the stomach.
d is secreted from the parietal cells lining the esophagus.

5. Pepsin

a helps to produce small peptide fragments.
b is secreted by parietal cells lying in the gastric pits in the fundus of the stomach.
c produces amino acids which are the major chemical stimuli for controlling pancreatic secretion.

6. Gastric secretion

a consists primarily of a basic solution (pH > 7.0) before food reaches the stomach.
b of HCl is increased by increased levels of gastrin.
c of gastrin is stimulated by protein in the stomach.
d is inhibited when there is fat in the duodenum.

Module III: Pancreatic Secretions; Secretion of Bile

Objectives

Upon completion of this module the student will be able to:

1. Contrast the exocrine and endocrine functions of the pancreas.
2. Name the two exocrine secretions of the pancreas; state their role in digestion.
3. Describe the cephalic, gastric, and intestinal phases of pancreatic secretions.
4. List the two hormones secreted from the duodenum that directly affect the pancreas and identify the effects they have on gastric motility, gastric secretions, and pancreatic secretions.
5. Identify the sites of formation and storage of bile.
6. List the primary constituents of bile.
7. Describe the factors that control bile secretion.
8. Describe the role of the enterohepatic circulation in bile recycling.

Reading Assignment

Chap. 12, pp. 373–379.

Exercises

Part I

Directions: Place an up (↑) or down (↓) arrow in each of the boxes in Fig. W-56 (p. 156) to indicate an increase or decrease in the rate of secretion.

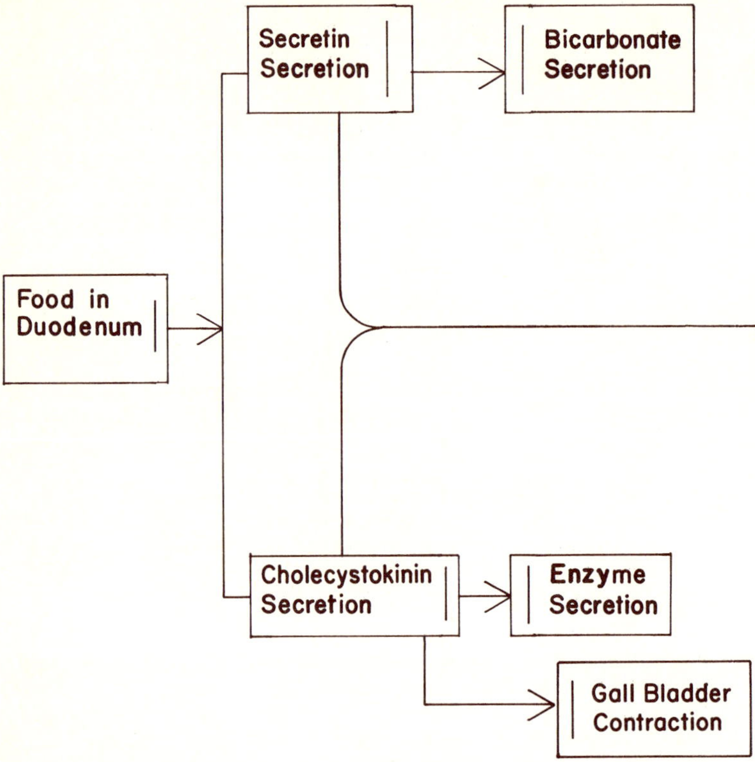

Fig. W-56 Process of pancreatic secretion.

Part II

Directions: Fill in the blanks in the following sentences with the missing words.

The F.B.I. Story—Part III

As you will remember from the previous module, G. I. George, physician, and friends are waiting in the hospital emergency room. George and Harold (the physician) have gotton to be great buddies during the two hours they have waited thus far—they are both fans of Mama's pizza and the New York Mets. George suggests that, as long as they are waiting, Harold might as well do a complete physical examination on him just for the fun of it. Harold agrees and begins work. After pinching and poking George for only a minute, Harold begins to probe George's gut, at which point George lets out a yelp. Harold announces that George seems to be having some trouble with his pancreatic or bile secretions, perhaps caused by gallstones (or the microfilm). After a good deal of investigation, Harold concludes that the pancreas is neutralizing the HCl secreted into the stomach at a normal rate. Eager to demonstrate his expertise, he explains to George and friends the process involved in neutralizing the stomach acid. What does he say?____________________ *(374)*

____

Since neutralization of stomach acid appears to be progressing normally, Harold assumes that the two hormones secreted by the duodenum that directly affect the pancreas are also moving along at a normal rate. What are the names of the two hormones that Harold is considering?

a ______________________________

b ______________________________ (375)

What effect do these hormones have on

a gastric motility? ______________________________

b gastric secretions? ______________________________

c pancreatic secretions? ______________________________ (375–376)

After verifying his assumptions, Harold turns his attention to the process of bile secretion. He begins by identifying the following things:

a site of formation of bile ______________________________

a site of storage of bile ______________________________

c four primary constituents of bile ______________________________

______________________________ (376)

Since George left Mama's Parlor only a short time ago (5:45 P.M., to be exact) Harold concludes that the cephalic phase of gastric secretion has already passed. Describe to George the stimuli (cephalic) for the release of bile. (378–379)

By this time, the intestinal stimuli for the release of bile should be at work. Describe to George the stimuli for this phase of bile secretion. (379)

After a bit more poking about, Harold determines that all of George's systems are "go" and that the pain George felt during the first part of the examination resulted from an anchovy protesting against being crushed in with the rest of the Heartburn Special. Again, George, Harold, and friends sit down to wait for the delivery of the microfilm.

See the next module for the conclusion of this exciting adventure story of the F.B.I.

Self-Test

Part I

Directions: Complete the following items in the space provided.

1. Describe the mechanism that controls the cephalic phase of pancreatic secretions.

2. Increased release of secretin and CCK has what effect upon the following?

a pancreatic secretions ______________________________

b gastric motility ______________________________

c gastric secretions ______________________________

3. On the chart below, list the two hormones released by the duodenum that directly affect pancreatic secretions, and identify the effect they have on the pancreas.

Hormones Affecting Pancreatic Secretions	Effects on Pancreas
1. ______________________	1. ______________________
	______________________
	______________________
2. ______________________	2. ______________________
	______________________
	______________________

4. Where is bile

   a stored? ______________________________

   b formed? ______________________________

5. George Peabody has a common case of "acid indigestion." In other words, his stomach is releasing an excess amount of HCl. What is George's pancreas doing in response to the increased acidity in his duodenum?

6. List the primary constituents of bile.

   a ______________________________

   b ______________________________

   c ______________________________

   d ______________________________

Part II

Directions: Circle the number of each item below that is *true*.

1. The pancreas helps to neutralize excess HCl released from the stomach by causing release of bicarbonate ions into the duodenal lumen.
2. Secretion of cholecystokinin is inhibited by the presence of fat molecules in the duodenum.
3. Increased release of bile may be caused by an emotional state brought on by the sight or smell of food.

Module IV: Small and Large Intestine

Objectives

Upon completion of this module, the student will be able to:

1. Describe motility of the intestine and the factors that affect it.
2. Identify the results of activity of the gastroileal reflex and the intestino-intestinal reflexes.
3. Describe the secretions of the small intestine.
4. Label on a diagram of the intestinal villus the following structures: microvilli, capillaries, arteries and arterioles, veins and venules, lacteal duct, and lymph duct.
5. Identify the functions of an intestinal villus.
6. Describe the digestion and absorption of carbohydrates, proteins, and fats in the intestine.
7. List the components of chyme in the large intestine.
8. List the substances that are absorbed or secreted by the large intestines.
9. Define *mass movement;* describe its role in the initiation of defecation.
10. Describe the process of defecation by listing the three major steps that occur during the process: contraction of the rectum, relaxation of internal and external anal sphincters, and increased peristaltic activity in the sigmoid colon.
11. State at least one fallacy noted in the text regarding constipation.
12. Describe the experimental evidence indicating that the symptoms accompanying constipation are the result of pressure in the rectum and colon.

Reading Assignment

Chap. 12, pp. 379–390.

Supplementary Materials

Information on the gastrocolic reflex: Distention of the stomach by food initiates contraction of the rectum and frequently a desire to defecate. (This reflex often occurs after a meal.)

Exercises

Part I

Directions: Complete the following items in the space provided. The result will be a brief description of the process of defecation and the conditions under which it occurs. See p. 389 for help.

1. The stimulus for defecation is usually the ______________________________ (2 words) of the fecal material into the rectum.
2. The stimulus causes sudden distention of the walls of the

______________________________.

3. The two occurrences above initiate the defecation reflex which is mediated primarily by the ______________________________ (3 words).
4. This reflex consists of ______________ of the rectum and relaxation of the ______________ and ______________ anal sphincters.
5. There is also increased ______________________________ (2 words) in the colon.
6. At this point, feces are propelled through the ______________________________.
7. Defecation is normally assisted by the following conditions:

   a ______________________________

   b ______________________________

   c ______________________________

Part II

The F.B.I. Story—Conclusion

After about four hours of waiting in the emergency room (it is now 9:42 P.M.) George excuses himself and repairs to the local men's room. He becomes very familiar with the process described in Part I of the Exercises in this module. (If *you* are not familiar with Part I of the Exercises, return to it and complete it now.) The results of the process are rushed by Harold to the lab for immediate examination. The lab technician quickly provides the small piece of microfilm and decontaminates it for George. Triumphant, he rushes back to the emergency room. Hilda is ecstatic. Hilda thanks George and Harold, and exits swiftly with the microfilm. Harold takes George aside. "Just as a matter of interest," says Harold, "what was on that film that was so all-fired important?"

"I am sworn to secrecy," says George, "but for a fellow fan of Mama's pizza and the New York Mets, I would do anything—well, almost anything. The film contains classified material that Hilda needs very badly before tomorrow morning. You see, she is taking a course in physiology. The film contains supplementary reading on the gastrocolic reflex that she needs to do before she can take the self-test on the small and large intestine."

Self-Test

Part I

Directions: Complete the following items in the space provided.

1. The major mechanism of intestinal motility is

   ____

2. List below three substances absorbed from the colon.

   a ______________________________

   b ______________________________

   c ______________________________
3. Describe the process of fat digestion and absorption.

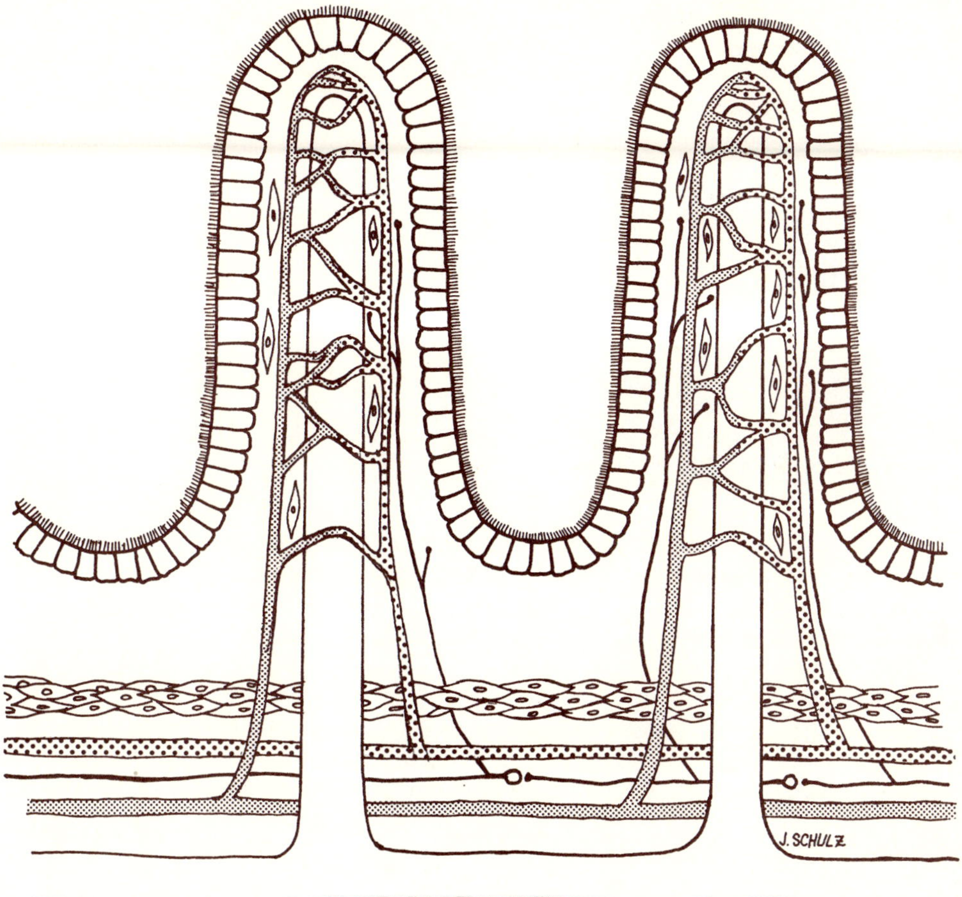

Fig. W-57

Part II

Directions: On Fig. W-57, a diagram of intestinal villi, label the following structures:

a microvilli
b capillaries
c arteries and arterioles
d veins and venules
e lacteal duct
f lymph duct

Part III

Directions: Circle the correct answer(s).

1. Miss Dental Health of 1976 has just finished eating a seven-course meal. Which of the following is happening in her intestines as she goes dutifully off to brush her pearly whites?

a Contractile activity in the ileum increases.
b Excitation of receptors in the stomach relates messages to the intestine.
c Segmentation occurs at a faster rate in the duodenum than in the ileum.
d The gastroileal reflex is stimulated.

2. The small intestinal villus

a has microvilli.
b is the structure that increases the surface area available for carrying out absorption.
c is covered with epithelial cells.
d moves in a rhythmic pattern that is the same as the basic electrical rhythm of the stomach.

3. Digestion

a of starch is carried out by amylase in the small intestine.
b for protein begins in the pancreas.
c of 50 percent of fat occurs in the stomach.
d of protein is assisted by proteolytic enzymes.

4. Constipation

a is the condition that exists when defecation occurs only at prolonged intervals.
b may occur when a person does not eat enough cellulosic (or bulk) material.
c when occurring for over 24 hr is harmful.
d symptoms include headache, nausea, and loss of appetite.

Module I:
The Absorptive and Postabsorptive States

Module II:
Insulin

Module III:
Epinephrine, Glucagon and Growth Hormone

Module IV:
Control of Growth

Module V:
Bioenergetics

Module VI:
Temperature Regulation

REGULATION OF ORGANIC METABOLISM AND ENERGY BALANCE

CHAPTER 13

Module I: The Absorptive and Postabsorptive States

Objectives

Upon completion of this module, the student will be able to:

1. Define *essential nutrient, molecular interconvertibility,* and *dynamic steady state.*
2. Identify the following as characteristics of carbohydrate, fat, and amino acid catabolism. (*a*) The major fate of both fat and carbohydrate is catabolism to yield energy, whereas amino acids can supply energy only after they are converted to carbohydrate or fat. (*b*) Excess carbohydrate and fat can be stored as such, whereas excess amino acids are not stored as protein but are converted to fat and carbohydrate.
3. Diagram the major inputs and outputs of the protein, carbohydrate, and fat pools (as in Fig. 13-1, p. 392, and Fig. 13-4, p. 394).
4. Diagram or list all major events of the absorptive period with regard to the processing of ingested carbohydrate, fat, and protein.
5. Describe the roles played by glucose in the liver in fat synthesis.
6. Diagram or list all the major events of the postabsorptive period in terms of blood glucose regulation.
7. Define *gluconeogenesis.*
8. Identify the changes occurring in the brain metabolism during prolonged fasting and the significance of these changes in terms of body functioning.

Reading Assignment

Chap. 13, pp. 391–398.

Exercises

Part I

Directions: Complete Fig. W-58 (p. 165), a diagram of carbohydrate and fat metabolism, by drawing arrows on the connecting lines to indicate direction of flow. (*394*)

Part II

Directions: Complete Fig. W-59 (p. 166), a diagram of protein metabolism, by drawing arrows on the connecting lines to indicate direction of flow. (*392*)

Part III

Directions: Complete the following items in the space provided.

1. Karl has just finished eating a sandwich furnished by one of the campus vending machines. It has been determined in previous studies that the bread from these

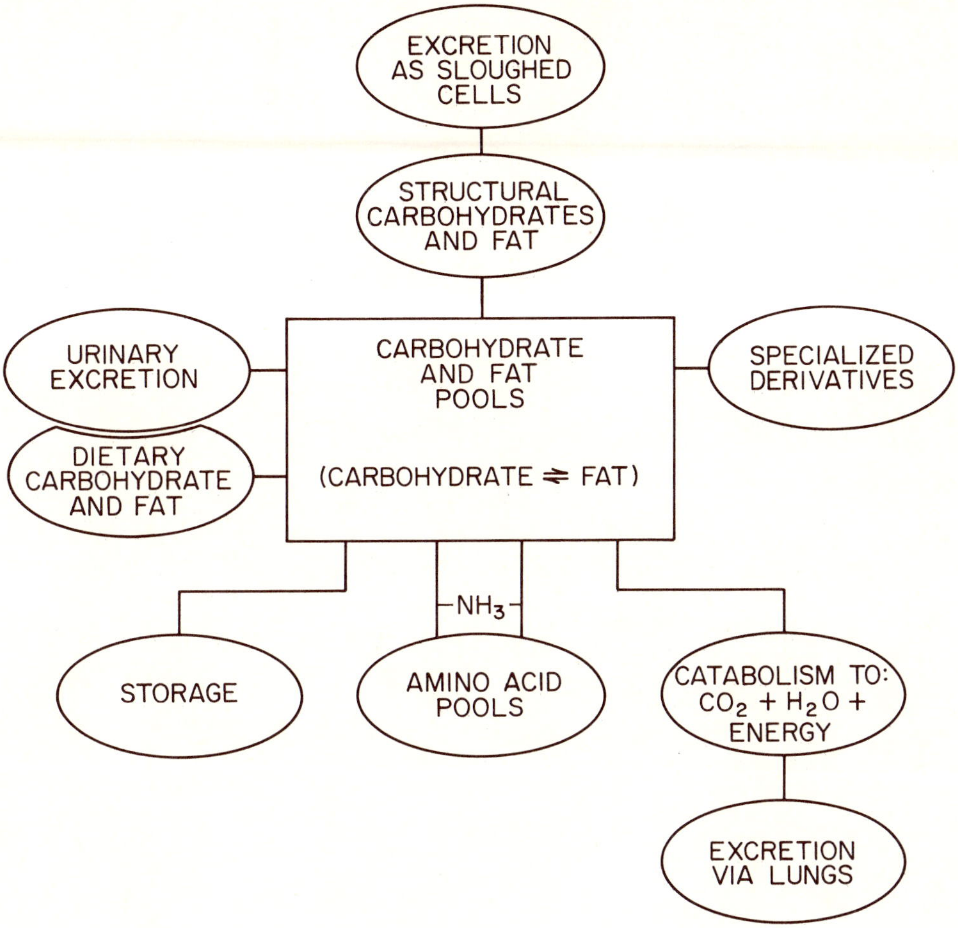

Fig. W-58 Carbohydrate and fat metabolism.

sandwiches is a pure form of carbohydrate. Assuming Karl ate only the bread from the sandwich, would you expect him to absorb into his blood all of the ingested carbohydrate in the form of glucose? ______________________________ (394)

2. Once into the blood, the absorbed monosaccharides pass through the ______________________________. (394)
3. The cells in the liver into which the carbohydrate is absorbed will convert the carbohydrate into ______________________________. (394)
4. In fact, there are three things that may happen to the bread ingested by Karl. Carbohydrates may

   a remain in the blood until synthesized into fat by the

   ______________________________,

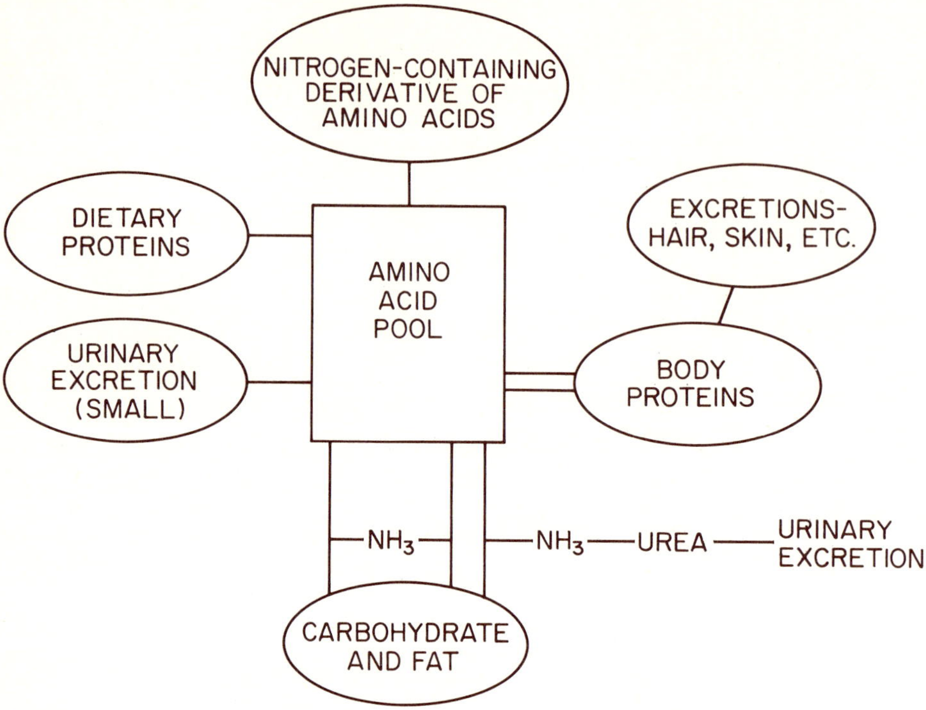

Fig. W-59 Protein metabolism.

b be stored as glycogen in the ______________________ or

______________________, or

c enter the cells of the body and be ______________________ for energy. (394)

5. Suppose Karl ate only the cheese (containing large amounts of fat) from his sandwich.

   a Is the fat absorbed into the blood (as are carbohydrates)?

   ______________________ (394)

   b Where are triglycerides (TG) stored? ______________________ (394)

6. Identify two sources of adipose tissue TG available in the body.

   a ______________________

   b ______________________ (394)

7. Is it possible that some of Karl's adipose tissue TG would be oxidized for energy for a postlunch basketball game? ______________________ (395)

8. The one slice of meat in Karl's sandwich would have many possible fates (assuming it contained pure amino acids). Many of the absorbed amino acids have the NH_3 portion of the molecule removed, thus becoming ______________________. (395)

9. What happens to the removed NH_3 portion of the molecule?

____ (395)

10. The keto acids that enter the Krebs tricarboxylic acid cycle provide energy for what cells? ______________________ (395)

11. Keto acids may also participate in fat synthesis by the liver by being converted into ______________________. (395)

12. Any amino acids not absorbed by the liver enter the ______________________. (395–396)

Self-Test

Part I

Directions: Complete the following items in the space provided or circle the correct answer(s).

1. During fasting, blood glucose may be available from

   a the liver only. *b* muscle only.
   c triglycerides only. *d* all three.

2. During long periods of fasting, the major source of blood glucose is ______________________

   ____.

3. During prolonged fasting,

   a body processes alter so as to preserve the plasma glucose level.
   b ketone bodies are formed.
   c the liver uses amino acids for energy.
   d gluconeogenesis takes place.

4. Describe the roles played by both the liver and glucose in fat synthesis.

5. Which of the following occurs during the absorptive phase of digestion?

   a Glucose provides the major source of energy.
   b A large percentage of the amino acids, fats, and carbohydrates are transformed into adipose tissue fat.
   c Many amino acids enter the liver where they are converted to glycerophosphate and ammonia.
   d Ammonia is converted to urea in the kidneys.

Part II

Directions: Complete Fig. W-60 (p. 168), a diagram of carbohydrate and fat metabolism, by writing the missing elements of the system in the empty boxes.

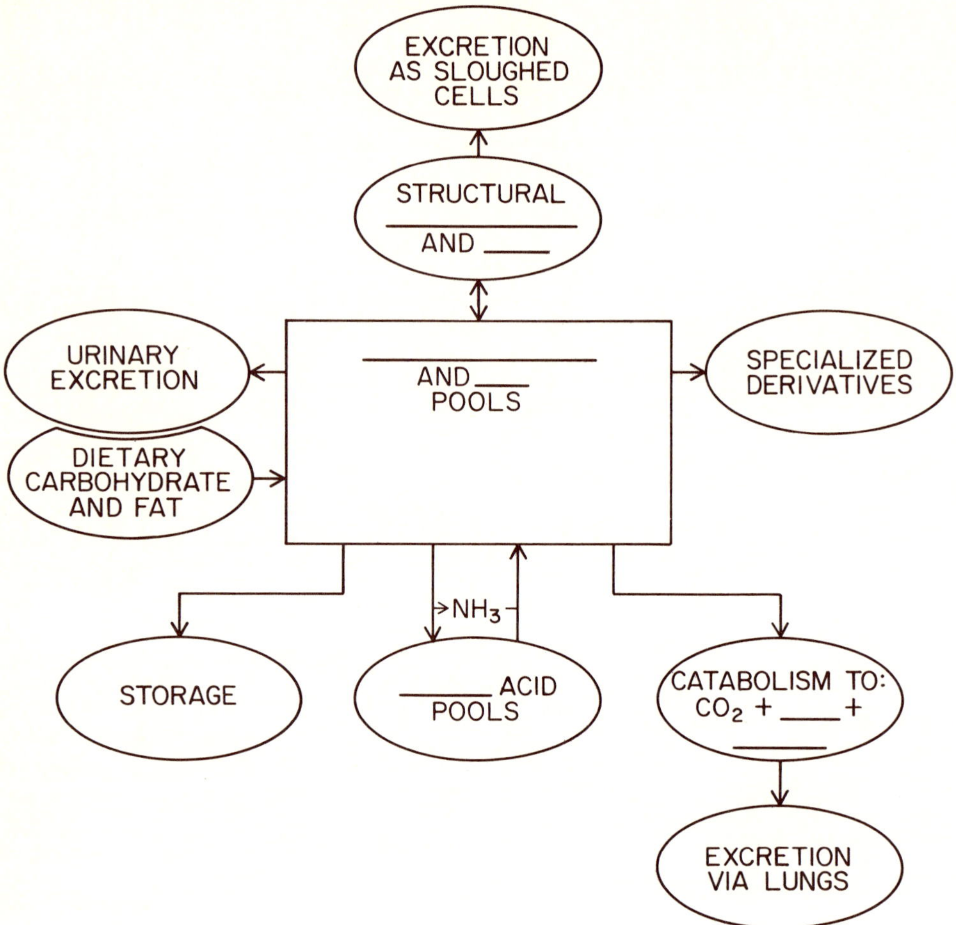

Fig. W-60

Module II: **Insulin**

Objectives

Upon completion of this module, the student will be able to:

1. Identify the site of production of insulin.
2. Describe the effect insulin has on glucose by identifying the mechanism controlling glucose uptake, and by identifying the major tissue which is not affected by insulin.

3. List the other direct effects insulin has on the human body in addition to its role in glucose uptake.
4. Identify the controls of the *rate* of insulin secretion.
5. State the effects of insulin deficit.
6. Describe the metabolic events occurring in a person who has diabetes mellitus.
7. Describe and explain the renal function and respiratory state of a patient with diabetes mellitus.

Reading Assignment

Chap. 14, pp. 398–402.

Supplementary Materials

Glucose-Tolerance Test

The glucose-tolerance test is used in the clinical diagnosis of diabetes. Administration of 1.75 g/kg glucose to a normal patient will cause a rise in blood glucose to approximately 140 mg/100 ml of blood. In a diabetic patient, the blood glucose levels could rise above 200 or 300 mg/100 ml. A patient with excess secretion of insulin will have an abnormally low initial blood sugar level as well as a lower peak following administration of glucose.

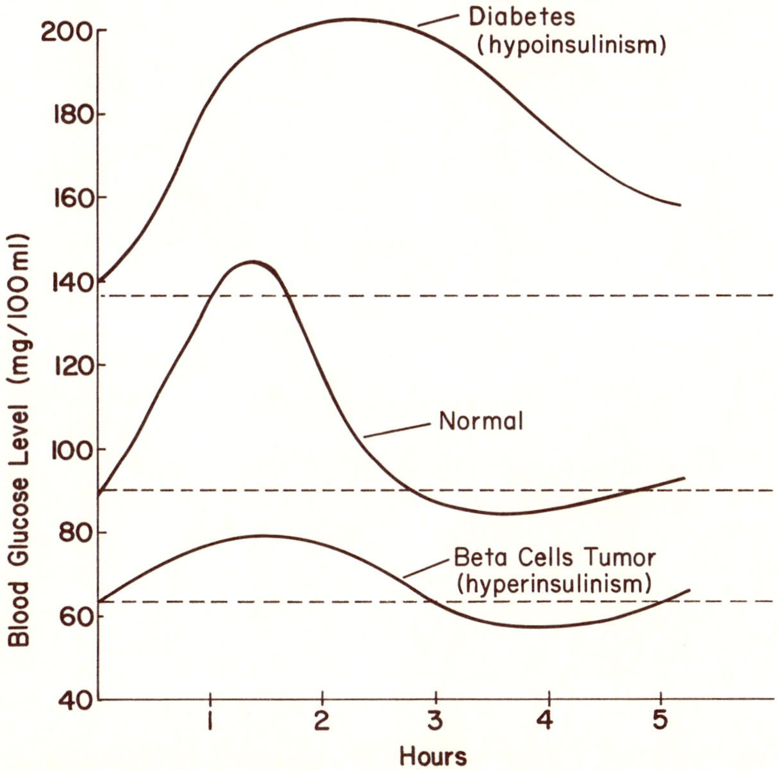

Fig. W-61 Glucose tolerance test.

Exercises

Directions: Complete the following items in the space provided or circle the correct answer(s).

1. George is currently undergoing tests to determine whether he has diabetes mellitus. Which of the following are symptoms that would cause his physician to check for diabetes?

   a weight gain despite reduced food intake
   b high plasma-glucose level
   c low plasma-glucose level
   d high volume of urine excreted
   e signs of "sugar" in the urine
   f signs of excess sodium in the urine (*399–402*)

2. What protein hormone is deficient in George (assuming he has diabetes mellitus)?

   ______________________________ (*401*)

3. Where is this hormone produced? ______________________________ (*398*)

4. Insulin deficiency in a person having diabetes mellitus causes (increased/decreased)

   permeability of cells to glucose. ______________________________ (*399*)

5. George demonstrates a marked increase in ventilation. Why does this increase in ventilation occur in persons who have diabetes mellitus? (*401*)

6. George's physician ordered a glucose-tolerance test (GTT) to help determine George's condition. Two tests got mixed up in the lab. Assuming George *does* have diabetes, which of the two tests shown in Fig. W-62 belongs to George? ________ (suppl.)

Self-Test

Part I

Directions: Circle T for true and F for false.

T F 1. Insulin is secreted by clusters of beta cells in the pancreas.
T F 2. Secretion of insulin is inhibited by elevations in plasma glucose levels.
T F 3. The rate of insulin secretion is controlled primarily by the glucose level of the blood flowing through the pancreas.
T F 4. A lowered concentration of insulin in the blood causes increased permeability of cells to glucose.
T F 5. A person who has untreated diabetes mellitus will most likely have increased ventilation.
T F 6. The brain's uptake of glucose is not dependent upon insulin.

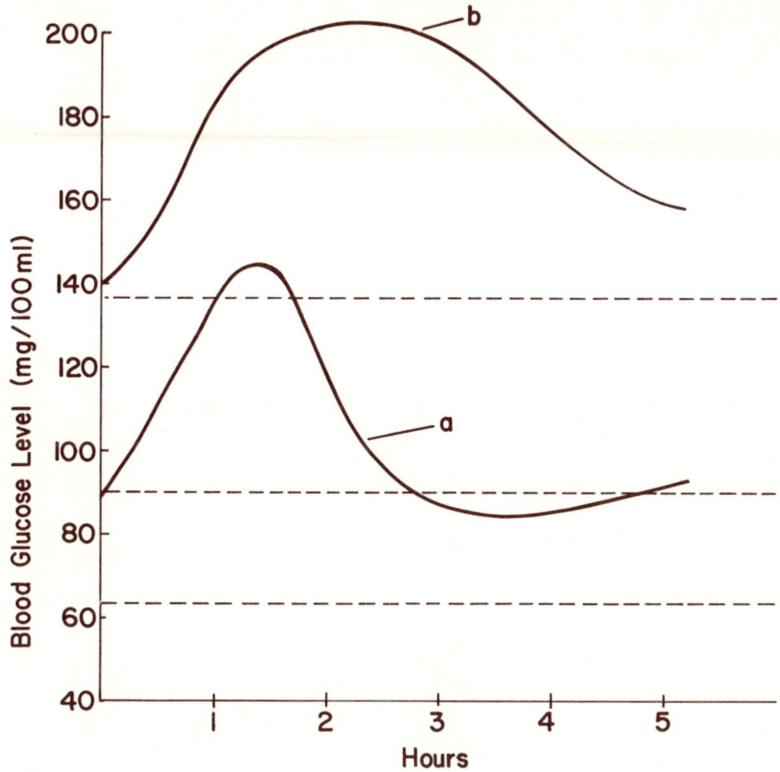

Fig. W-62 Abnormal and normal GTT.

Part II

Directions: Circle the correct answer(s).

1. Which of the following are stimulated directly or indirectly by insulin?

   a glucose synthesis *b* glycogen synthesis
   c fat synthesis *d* glucose oxidation

2. In a person having untreated diabetes mellitus, lowered insulin concentration causes

   a catabolism of triglycerides into fatty acids and ketone bodies.
   b the absorptive state to operate continually.
   c weight gain.
   d all of these.

3. In the kidney of a person having untreated diabetes mellitus

   a glucose may exceed its T_m and be excreted in the urine.
   b ketone bodies and glucose in the urine create an osmotic diuresis.
   c sodium reabsorption is retarded.
   d in response to the elevation in H^+, the kidneys excrete excess HCO_3^-.

Module III: Epinephrine, Glucagon, and Growth Hormone

Objectives

Upon completion of this module, the student will be able to:

1. Describe the control and site of secretion of epinephrine, glucagon, and growth hormone.
2. Describe the actions of epinephrine, glucagon, and growth hormone on carbohydrate and lipid metabolism (see Table 13-1, p. 403).
3. State the effects of a high-protein meal on insulin, glucagon, and growth hormone.
4. State the role of growth hormone, epinephrine, and glucagon in stress.
5. Differentiate between glycogenolysis and gluconeogenesis.

Reading Assignment

Chap. 13, pp. 402–406.

Exercises

Part I

Directions: Complete the following items in the space provided.

1. List at least three effects epinephrine has on organic metabolism in general.

   a ______________________________

   b ______________________________

   c ______________________________ (*403*)

2. Describe the control of release of epinephrine. (*403*)

3. Where is glucagon produced? ______________________________ (*402*)
4. List the three metabolic events stimulated by glucagon.

   a ______________________________

   b ______________________________

   c ______________________________ (*403*)

5. Is plasma glucose concentration higher during the absorptive or the postabsorptive state? ______________________ (403)

6. Name the direct control of glucagon secretion. ______________________
______________________ (403)

7. Identify the four effects GH has on organic metabolism.
   a ______________________
   b ______________________
   c ______________________
   d ______________________ (403–404)

8. Describe the neuroendocrine pathway by which GH secretion is altered. (404–405)

9. Indicate whether GH secretion increases, decreases, or remains the same in each of the following situations.
   a during eating ______________________
   b during fasting ______________________
   c under stress ______________________ (403–405)

10. Identify the direct control of GH secretion. ______________________
______________________ (405)

11. Indicate whether plasma glucose concentration increases or decreases after administration of each of the following substances.
   a insulin ______________________
   b glucagon ______________________
   c epinephrine ______________________
   d growth hormone ______________________ (406)

Part II

Directions: Complete Chart 1 (p. 174). List the hormones insulin, glucagon, growth hormone, and epinephrine in their proper location. (399–403)

Chart 1

Metabolic Variable	Increased By	Decreased By
Glucose uptake		
Glycogen storage (glycogenesis)		
Adipose tissue TG storage		
Plasma glucose concentration		
Plasma fatty-acid concentration		
Liver gluconeogenesis		

Self-Test

Part I

Directions: Circle T for true and F for false.

T F 1. Epinephrine stimulates glycogen breakdown in liver and muscle.
T F 2. Epinephrine inhibits breakdown of triglycerides in adipose tissue.
T F 3. Hypoglycemia causes increased release of epinephrine.
T F 4. Glucagon is produced by alpha cells in the islets of Langerhans.
T F 5. Plasma glucose concentration is higher during the postabsorptive period.
T F 6. Glucagon secretion is controlled by plasma glucose level.
T F 7. Growth hormone (GH) inhibits uptake and oxidation of glucose by many tissues of the body.
T F 8. Growth hormone (GH) tends to stimulate adipose tissue breakdown.
T F 9. During fasting, GH secretion remains elevated.
T F 10. GH secretion is controlled by the plasma pH.
T F 11. Administration of insulin would tend to make the concentration of plasma glucose go up.

Part II

Directions: Circle the correct answer(s).

1. Plasma GH will increase upon administration of

   a insulin. *b* glucagon.
   c epinephrine. *d* all three.

2. GH secretion increases during

   a eating of a normal, well-balanced meal.
   b fasting over two days' time.
   c administration of glucagon.
   d times of extreme stress.

3. Glucagon secretion

   a leads to increased gluconeogenesis.
   b results in increased glycogenesis.
   c is increased during the postabsorptive state.
   d is stimulated by a lowered plasma glucose concentration.

Module IV: Control of Growth

Objectives

Upon completion of this module, the student will be able to:

1. Differentiate between true growth and a simple gain in weight.
2. Define *critical period of development.*
3. State the relation between an individual's growth capacity and environmental (external) factors.
4. Describe the metabolic effects of growth hormone on growth.
5. Describe thyroxine's effects on growth.
6. Describe the effect of androgens and estrogens on general body growth.
7. Define *compensatory hypertrophy;* give an example.

Reading Assignment

Chap. 13, pp. 406–410.

Exercises

Part I

Directions: Complete the following items in the space provided.

1. A normal amount of thyroxin is necessary for normal growth. Will administration of excess thyroxin lead to excess growth? What will be its effect?

2. Describe the possible effects resulting from deficient thyroid activity during growth. *(407–409)*

Part II

Directions: Describe what Fig. W-63 (p. 176) tells you about critical periods of growth and the possible results of temporary malnutrition. *(406)*

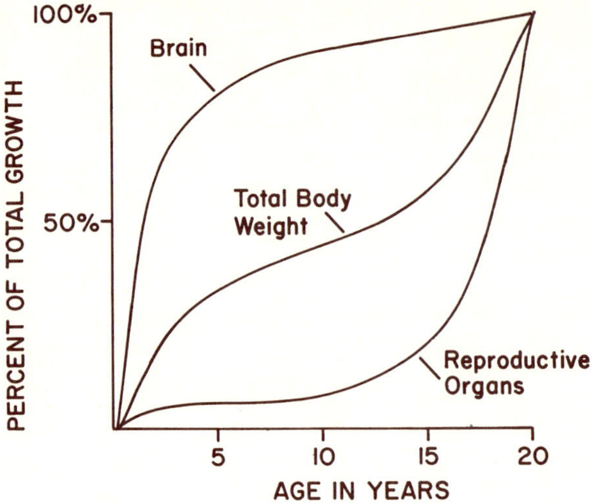

Fig. W-63

Self-Test

Part I

Directions: Circle T for true and F for false.

T F 1. The critical period of development occurs during the same period of time for all tissues.

T F 2. Part of thyroxin's effect is to promote the effect of growth hormone.

T F 3. Androgens and estrogens stimulate protein synthesis only in the reproductive organs.

T F 4. It is trauma to the neural innervation to an organ which appears to stimulate compensatory hypertrophy of that organ.

Part II

Directions: Circle the correct answer(s).

1. Hormone(s) that act(s) to stop bone growth by inducing conversion of the epiphyseal plates is (are)

   a growth hormone. *b* thyroxin.
   c androgens. *d* glucagon.

2. Acromegaly results from an increase in hormone(s) after loss of the cartilage in long bones. The hormone(s) responsible is (are)

   a growth hormone. *b* thyroxin.
   c androgens. *d* estrogen.

3. The hormone(s) whose deficiency results in a failure of nerve myelination is (are)

   a growth hormone. *b* thyroxin.
   c androgens. *d* estrogen.

4. The real criterion(ia) for defining true growth is (are)

   a increase in size.
   b increase in weight.
   c formation and elimination of waste products.
   d increased synthesis and accumulation of protein.
   e increased utilization of growth hormone.

Module V: Bioenergetics

Objectives

Upon completion of this unit the student will be able to:

1. State the first law of thermodynamics and apply the equation $\Delta E = \Delta$ heat $+ \Delta$ work to the concept of metabolic rate.
2. Distinguish between internal and external work.
3. Describe energy balance by stating the formula

   Total energy expenditure = heat produced + external work + energy storage

4. Define *metabolic rate;* state how it is measured.
5. Define *basal metabolic rate;* distinguish between the terms *metabolic rate* and *basal metabolic rate* (BMR).
6. Identify the appropriate units of measurement for BMR.
7. Define *metabolic cost of living* and *specific dynamic action.*
8. List the factors that influence metabolic rate; state the mechanisms by which they exert their effects.
9. State the overall energy balance formula as

   Food energy intake = heat produced + external work + energy storage

   and describe what happens when food intake is greater than or less than the total energy expenditure.
10. Describe the control of food intake by hypothalamic integrating centers by identifying the effects of stimulating or of destroying the midline portion and the outer hypothalamus.
11. List the signals that influence the hypothalamus centers involved in the control of food intake, including discussions of the glucostatic, lipostatic, and thermostatic theories, and the psychological factors.
12. Define *obesity* and name its ultimate cause.
13. Describe the interaction between diet and exercise in the maintenance of body weight.

Reading Assignment

Chap. 13, pp. 410–421.

Exercises

Directions: Answer the following questions in the space provided.

1. You are going to determine the basal metabolic rate (BMR) of a patient. Name at least three conditions that are necessary in order to determine the BMR. (*411–412*)

   a ______

   b ______

   c ______

2. Would the metabolic rate of the same subject when not in the postabsorptive state be higher or lower than above? (*412*)

   ______

   Why? ______

   ______

3. Suppose an individual has an inoperable tumor in the midline portion of the hypothalamus. What effect might this have on food intake? (*415*)

4. Write an equation for the total energy expenditure of the body (see p. 411). Under what conditions does food intake equal the internal heat production and external work? (*414*)

5. Briefly describe the theories concerning the signals which influence the hypothalamic centers involved in food intake. (*416–418*)

Self-Test

Part I

Directions: Circle the correct answer(s).

1. Which of these factors can significantly change the metabolic rate?

   a emotions　　*b* clothing
   c muscle tone　　*d* exercise
   e SDA　　*f* aging
   g surface area of body　　*h* pregnancy

2. A woman is approximately 50 pounds overweight. What else can be said for sure about this individual?

   a She has a lower metabolism than normal.
   b She eats more than the average person.
   c She has an emotional problem.
   d She has a poor heat-control mechanism.
   e She would be helped if the midline portion of her hypothalamus were destroyed, which would help her reduce by inhibiting her eating.
   f She is suffering from a hyperthyroidism.
   g Her normal food-intake control mechanisms have failed.
   h If she continued her present eating habits, she could still lose weight.

Part II

Directions: Answer the following questions in the space provided.

1. Write the formula that describes steady state energy balance (including food intake, metabolic heat production, and external work).

2. Write a brief definition of specific dynamic action.

3. Write the first law of thermodynamics as it relates to the human body.

4. Describe the indirect method for measuring metabolic rate.

Module VI: Temperature Regulation

Objectives

Upon completion of this unit, the student will be able to:

1. Identify the adaptive significance of homeothermy.
2. Describe the normal variations in body temperature.
3. Identify the physiological sources of heat production and the conditions under which storage of heat occurs.

4. Describe the mechanisms of heat loss, including a discussion of radiation, conduction, convection, sweating, and their relation to blood flow and to behavioral changes.
5. State how evaporation from the body surface and linings of the respiratory tract results in heat loss.
6. Identify the mechanisms allowing acclimation to high temperatures.
7. Describe the pathways of information which coordinate temperature regulation, including thermoreceptors (central and peripheral) and the hypothalamic integrating centers.
8. Identify the source and cause of fever.
9. Differentiate between heat stroke and heat exhaustion.

Reading Assignment

Chap. 13, pp. 421–429.

Exercises

Part I

Directions: Answer the following questions in the space provided.

1. What are the mechanisms that allow one to survive exposure to the cold? (426)

2. What are the mechanisms that allow one to survive exposure to heat? (426)

Part II

Directions: Supply the information needed to complete the following chart. Try to supply at least one example for each of the spaces. (426)

	Voluntary Behavior	Physiological Change
In response to cold:		
To decrease heat loss		
To increase heat production		
In response to heat:		
To increase heat loss		
To decrease heat production		

Part III

Directions: Answer the following items in the space provided.

1. What is the adaptive significance of homeothermy? (*421*)

2. Describe the thermoregulatory effects of warming or cooling the hypothalamus, or skin. (*427–428*)

Self-Test

Part I

Directions: Circle the correct answer(s).

1. On entering a cold environment
   a our peripheral blood vessels become vasoconstricted.
   b we decrease our production of sweat.
   c our muscle tone decreases.
   d our *basal* metabolic rate increases.
   e we increase our skin surface area.
2. In a hot environment
   a vasoconstriction of our skin blood vessels occurs.
   b after several days, our production of sweat has increased and the sodium content has decreased.
   c we voluntarily decrease our activity.
   d our hypothalamus receives information about the high environmental temperature from peripheral receptors in the skin.

Part II

Directions: Circle T for true and F for false.

T F 1. A desert nomad would have a higher salt content in his sweat than an Eskimo.
T F 2. As the external environmental temperature drops, reflexive controls increase peripheral vasoconstriction.
T F 3. A prostaglandin might lead to fever by causing a depression in the hypothalamic "set-point."
T F 4. Infections lead to the inability of the body to regulate its temperature, and thus cause fevers.
T F 5. Aspirin is an inhibitor of prostaglandin synthesis.

Module I:
Male Reproductive Physiology

Module II:
Female Reproductive Physiology

Module III:
Pregnancy

Module IV:
Birth Control, Sex Determination, Puberty, and Menopause

CHAPTER 14 REPRODUCTION

Module I: Male Reproductive Physiology

Objectives

Upon completion of this module, the student will be able to:

1. Define *gonad, ovary, testis, accessory reproductive organ, secondary sexual characteristics, puberty.*
2. Define *spermatogenesis.*
3. Name and describe the function of the two different tissues that make up the testes.
4. Describe the interdependence of spermatogenesis and testosterone.
5. Describe spermatogenesis, including the terms spermatogonia, primary spermatocyte, secondary spermatocyte, spermatid, and spermatozoa.
6. Contrast mitosis and meiosis in terms of location and numbers of chromosomes present after the final division.
7. Label the following items on a simplified diagram of the testes and other male reproductive structures, and give the function of each (see Figs. 14-1, 14-2, 14-5): seminiferous tubules, epididymis, vas deferens, prostate gland, seminal vesicles, bulbo-urethral (or Cowper's) gland, urethra, location of sertoli cells, interstitial cells, scrotum, and testes.
8. Identify the following areas on a diagram of the male reproductive structures (see Figs. 14-1, 14-2, 14-5): site of spermatogenesis, sperm storage site, site of a vasectomy (see supplementary materials), route of movement of sperm from testis to outside world, and site of testosterone production and secretion.
9. List the constituents of semen.
10. Describe the vascular mechanism for producing erection in the male; describe the vessels' neural control.
11. Define *impotence.*
12. Describe ejaculation; list the receptors, afferent and efferent pathways, site of the integrating center, effector organs, and reflex response.
13. Define *orgasm.*
14. Differentiate between erection, emission, and ejaculation.
15. Describe testosterone, its chemical nature, site of synthesis, sites and mechanism of action, effects, and stimuli for release.
16. Name the anterior pituitary gonadotropins that control testicular function; state their effects on spermatogenesis and testosterone secretion.
17. Describe the hypothalamic control of the pituitary gonadotropins.

Reading Assignment

Chap. 14, pp. 430–438.

Supplementary Materials

See Module IV supplementary materials for a discussion of vasectomy and tubal ligation.

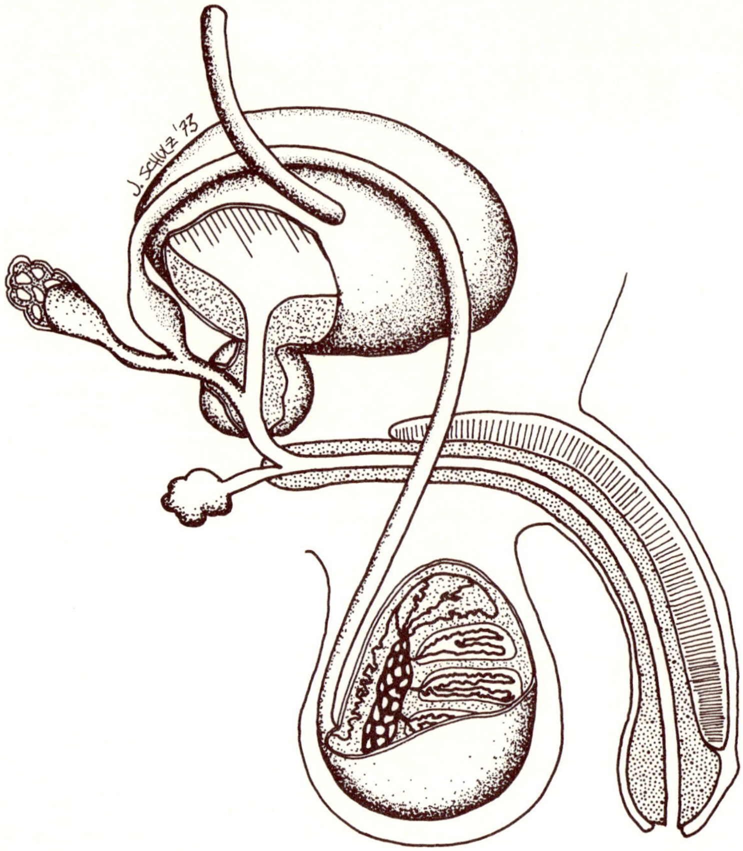

Fig. W-64 Male reproductive system.

Exercises

Part I

Directions: On Fig. W-64, label the following items.

a seminiferous tubules	*b* epididymis
c vas deferens	*d* seminal vesicles
e prostate gland	*f* bulbo-urcthral gland

(*434*)

Part II

Directions: Answer the following questions in the space provided.

1. Andrew (a male child) has low testosterone secretion. What would be the result of this condition if he had no treatment? (*436–437*)

2. Andrew's hormone condition was treated at an early age and his sexual development occurred at a natural rate. At the age of fifteen he began having erotic dreams that caused him to have erections. Describe the vascular mechanism and the neural control that made this possible. (*434–435*)

3. Andrew met Ann and they plan to be married. They each had a full physical examination and found they both have erratic hormones. The doctor's reports on Andrew and Ann follow. Complete the forms you think the doctor would have.

LAB REPORT

Name: Andrew Andrews Date: February 1, 1972

FINDINGS: EFFECT ON:

	High	Normal	Low	
Testosterone	X			1. Plasma LH: ________ ________________ (*437–438*)
				2. Sexual organs: ________ ________________ (*436*)
FSH			X	3. Spermatogenesis: ________ ________________ (*437–438*)

LAB REPORT

Name: Ann Drogen Date: February 1, 1972

FINDINGS: EFFECT ON:

X 1. High androgen level 1. Secondary sexual characteristics and fertility: ________

____

____

____

____

________________ (*437*)

Part III

Directions: Answer the following questions in the space provided.

1. Describe and compare the nervous pathways necessary for erection and ejaculation. *(434–435)*

2. What is the response of the skeletal muscle and of the smooth muscle of the ducts and blood vessels during ejaculation? *(435)*

Self-Test

Part I

Directions: On Fig. W-65, a diagram of the male testis, clearly label the following structures.

a seminiferous tubules *b* epididymis
c vas deferens *d* prostate

Using arrows, indicate the route of movement of sperm from testis to the outside of the body.

Part II

Directions: Circle the correct answer(s).

1. Increasing the testosterone in a female to a high level would, in time, cause
   - *a* sterility.
   - *b* enlarged breasts.
   - *c* growth of facial hair.
   - *d* enlargement of skeletal mass.
   - *e* enlargement of the clitoris.
   - *f* a lower-pitched voice.
2. The probable cause of deficient erection and ejaculation, decreased size in reproductive organs, and inhibition of the smooth muscle activities in the ducts in the male adult, would be
   - *a* increased LH secretion.
   - *b* high testosterone secretion.
   - *c* high FSH secretion.
   - *d* decreased spermatogenesis.
   - *e* castration.
   - *f* low testosterone secretion.
   - *g* increased spermatogenesis.
3. Low testosterone secretion in a male child at puberty would most likely result in
   - *a* an increase in LH secretion.
   - *b* decreased spermatogenesis.

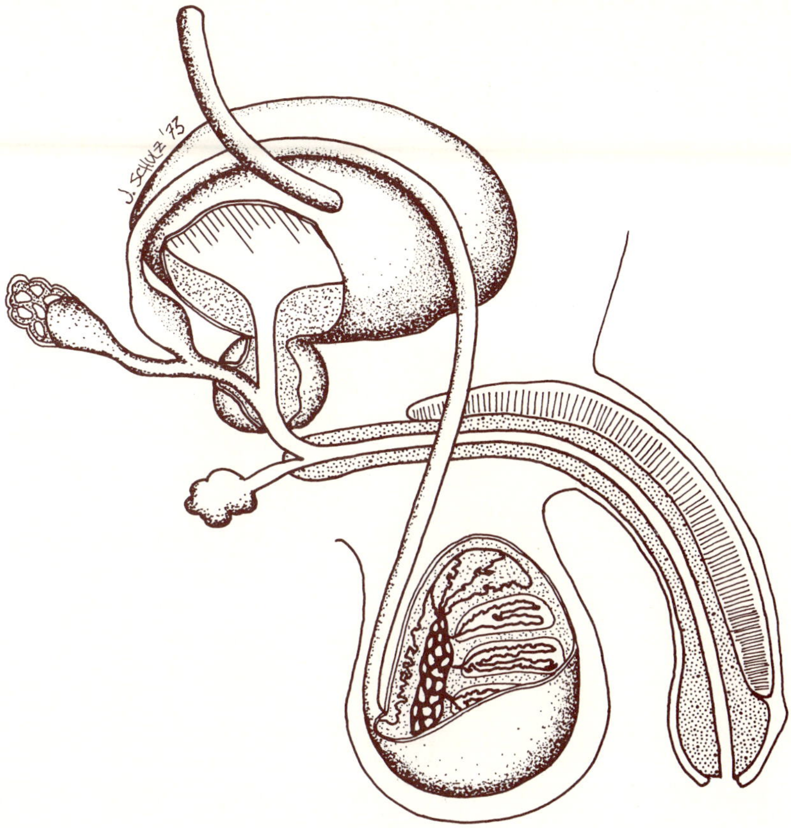

Fig. W-65

c inhibited development of the sex organs.
d female fat distribution.
e feminine behavior.

4. Low secretion of the luteinizing hormone (LH) in the normal male adult would cause

a inhibition of testosterone secretion.
b excessive beard growth.
c increased spermatogenesis.
d shrinkage of the anterior pituitary glands.

5. Increased testosterone secretion in the male causes

a decreased LH secretion.
b decreased FSH secretion.
c no changes at all.
d increased feminine behavior.
e shrinkage of the sex organs.
f increased LH secretion.

6. Erection of the penis in the male

   a is caused by the expansion of the erectile tissue.
   b cannot occur without stimulation of the mechanoreceptors at the tip of the penis.
   c is aided by the constriction of veins emptying the erectile chambers.
   d occurs when arterioles supplying the erectile chambers are constricted.

7. In the human male,

   a sperm are stored in the epididymis and in the first part of the vas deferens before ejaculation.
   b spermatogenesis occurs in the seminiferous tubules.
   c a vasectomy is performed to terminate spermatogenesis.
   d following castration, the accessory reproductive organs decrease in size.

8. Which of the following is (are) true of ejaculaton in the male?

   a It has an afferent pathway identical to that for erection.
   b Sperm are able to leak into the bladder.
   c It results from contraction of smooth muscle only.
   d It is followed by a latent period during which erection is impossible.

9. The term emission refers to

   a expelling of the semen from the penis.
   b movement of the genital duct contents into the urethra.
   c leakage of urine into the ejaculate.
   d movement of the contents of the seminiferous tubules into the epididymis.

Part III

Directions: Complete the following items in the space provided.

1. Ejaculation is usually accompanied by intense pleasure known as

   ______________________________.

2. During spermatogenesis, meiosis takes place between two specific stages. It occurs

   between the ______________________________ and

   the ______________________________.

3. Inability to obtain an erection is termed ______________________________.
4. Testosterone is produced by interstitial cells which are located

   ______________________________.

5. The major constituents of semen are ______________________________

   ______________________________.

Module II: Female Reproductive Physiology

Objectives

Upon completion of this module, the student will be able to:

1. Describe the following ovarian structures: primordial follicle, mature follicle, zona pellucida, antrum, and corpus luteum.
2. Describe the mitotic and meiotic divisions of the ovum; contrast oogenesis (ovum development) with spermatogenesis.
3. Name the ovarian hormones; state their chemical nature and site of origin.
4. Mark the follicular phase, the luteal phase, and the day of ovulation, on a scale of 28 days, beginning with day one as the first day of menstrual bleeding.
5. State the changes in LH, FSH, estrogen, and progesterone throughout the 28-day menstrual cycle; explain why these changes occur.
6. Describe the hormonal control of follicle and ovum development.
7. Describe the hormonal control of ovulation.
8. State the factors responsible for the LH peak in midcycle.
9. Describe the function of the corpus luteum.
10. Define *myometrium* and *endometrium*.
11. Identify the menstrual, proliferative, and secretory phases, on a 28-day scale, beginning with day one as the first day of menstrual bleeding.
12. Describe the changes in uterine endometrium during the menstrual cycle; explain them in terms of the hormonal patterns.
13. State the nonuterine effects of estrogen and progesterone (see Table 14-1, p. 447).
14. Describe the female sexual response as presented on p. 448.
15. Name the hormones controlling sex drive in the female.

Reading Assignment

Chap. 14, pp. 438–449.

Exercises

Part I

Directions: On Fig. W-66 (p. 190), a diagram of a woman's ovaries, label the following items.

a mature follicle
b ovum
c site of secretion of estrogen (*440*)

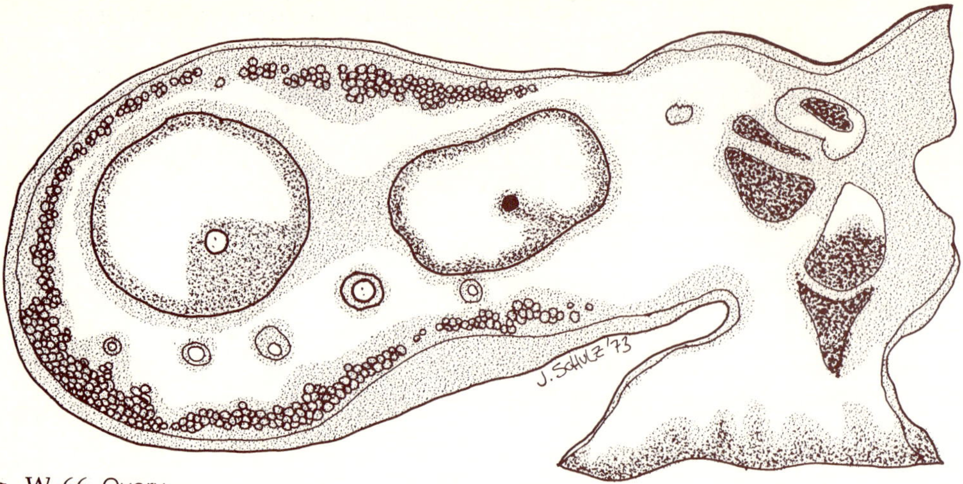

Fig. W-66 Ovary.

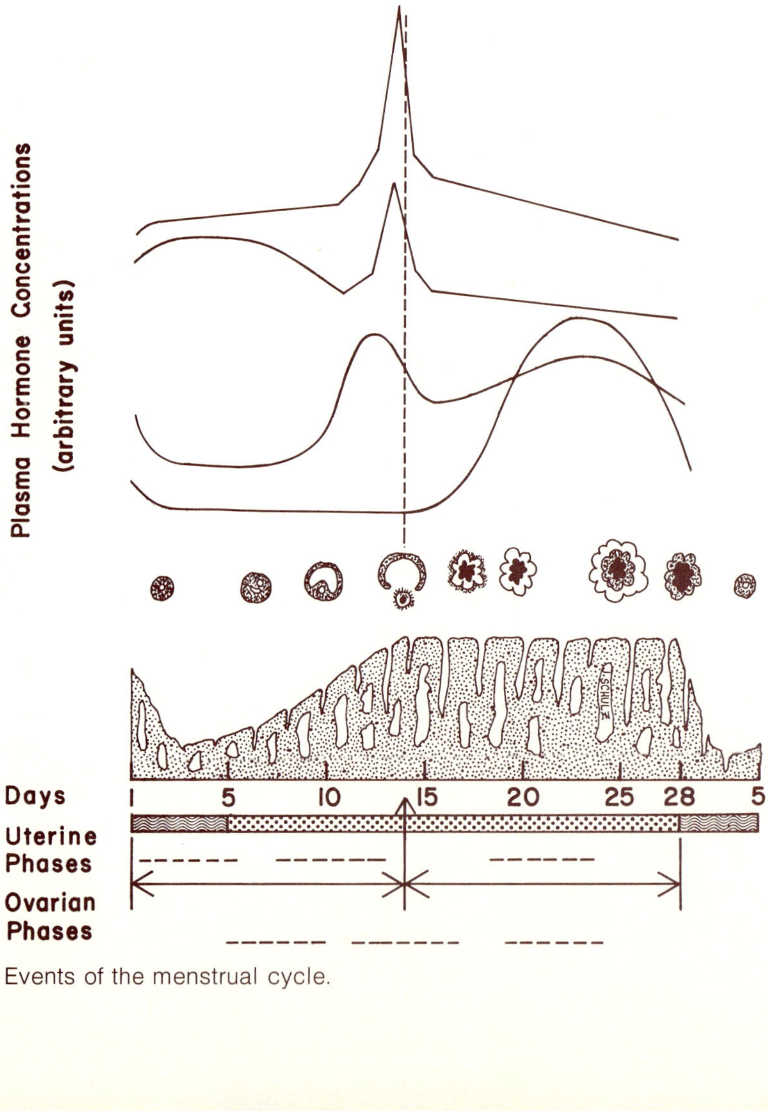

Fig. W-67 Events of the menstrual cycle.

Part II

Directions: Fig. W-67 shows the secretion patterns of a woman's hormones. Label the following items.

a LH pattern of fluctuation
b FSH pattern of fluctuation
c secretion patterns of estrogen
d secretion patterns of progesterone
e follicular phase of the cycle
f the "fertile" period
g the point of ovulation
h luteal phase of cycle
i proliferative phase of the cycle
j secretory phase of the cycle *(443)*

Part III

Directions: Answer the following questions in the space provided.

1. Fill in the blanks in Fig. W-68.

    (1) ________________________________

    (2) ________________________________

    (3) ________________________________

    (4) ________________________________ *(445–446)*

2. Regarding the events depicted in Fig. W-68:

    a Describe the stages of ovum development (oogenesis). *(439–440)*

    b Describe the interaction of hormones which control the menstrual cycle. *(446)*

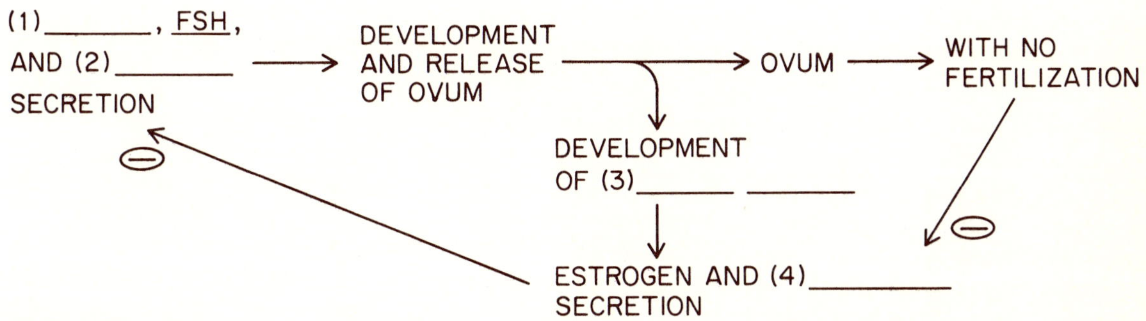

Fig. W-68

Self-Test

Part I

Directions: Circle the correct answer(s).

1. Ovulation results from a midcycle increase in

   a FSH. *b* LH.
   c estrogen. *d* progesterone.

2. Progesterone secretion is highest during which of the following phases?

   a follicular *b* luteal
   c proliferative *d* menstrual flow

3. Follicle and ovum development is dependent on the presence of

   a FSH. *b* LH.
   c estrogen. *d* progesterone.

4. A decrease in blood estrogen and progesterone levels resulting from degeneration of the corpus luteum leads to what endometrial changes?

   a proliferation *b* secretion
   c menstruation *d* blastocyst implantation

Part II

Directions: Circle T for true and F for false.

T F 1. Sex drive in the female is thought to be controlled mainly by blood levels of estrogen.
T F 2. Myometrium is the smooth muscle layer of the uterus.
T F 3. Progesterone is secreted in increasingly large amounts as the follicle develops.
T F 4. One important nonuterine effect of estrogen is the lowering of plasma cholesterol.
T F 5. It is the increase in progesterone near the end of the cycle that leads to menstruation.
T F 6. The thick membrane formed by the follicle cells between themselves and the ovum is termed the antrum.
T F 7. In contrast to spermatogenesis, during oogenesis each primitive ovum produces only one mature ovum containing 23 chromosomes.

Part III

Direction: Using Fig. W-69, a composite diagram of hormonal and other events in the menstrual cycle, label

a the point of ovulation.
b the LH pattern of fluctuation.
c the follicular phase of the cycle.
d the secretion pattern of estrogen.
e the secretion pattern of progesterone.
f the "fertile period" of the cycle.
g the FSH pattern of fluctuation.

Part IV

Directions: Using Fig. W-70, a simplified diagram of the ovary, label the site of estrogen secretion, mature follicle, ovum.

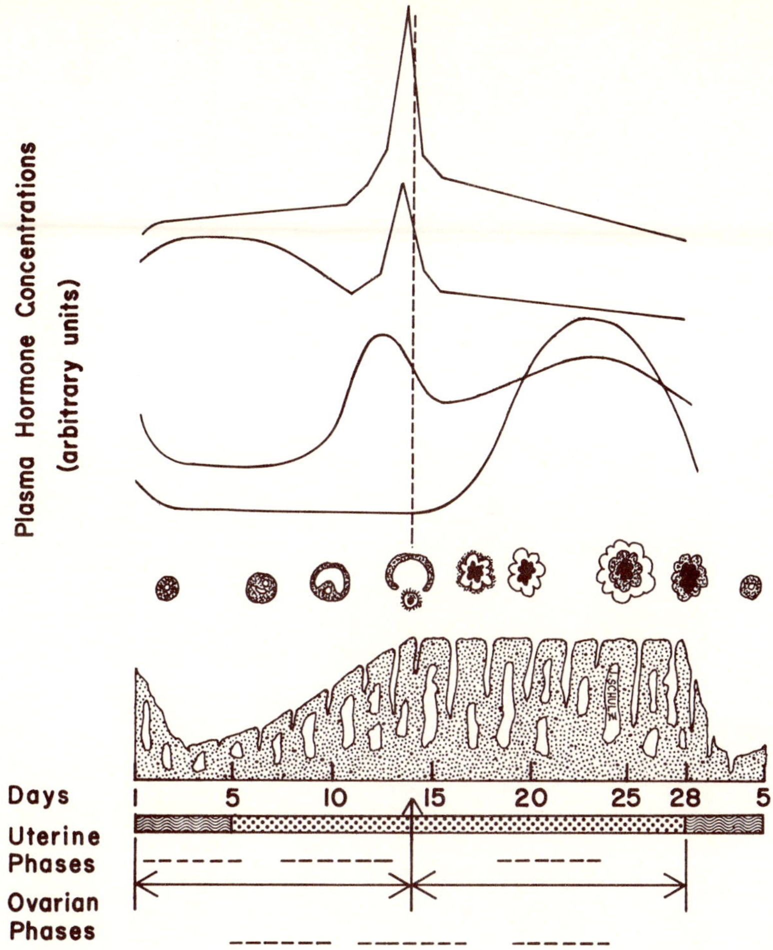

Fig. W-69

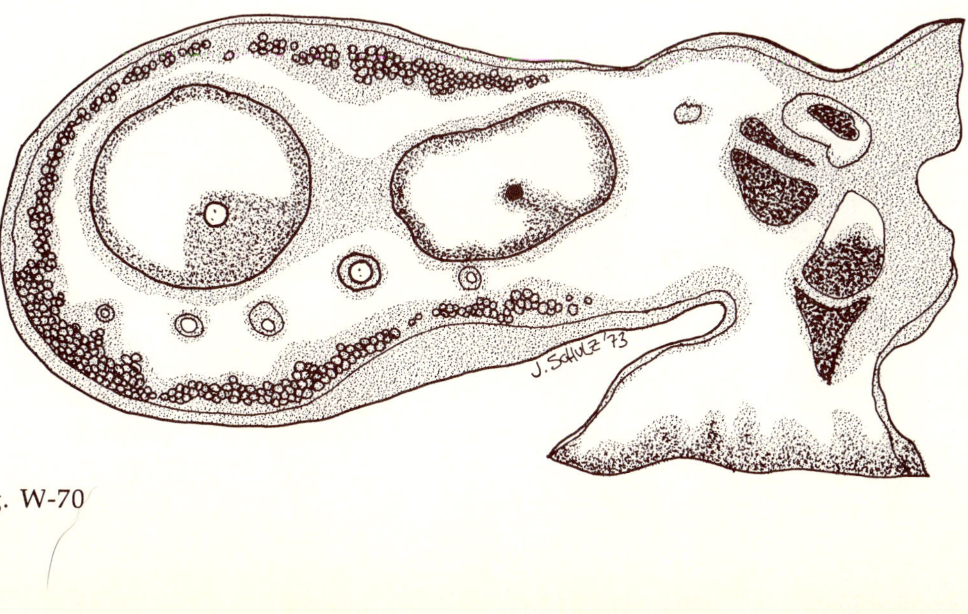

Fig. W-70

Module III: Pregnancy

Objectives

Upon completion of this module, the student will be able to:

1. State the duration of sperm and ovum viability after ejaculation or ovulation.
2. Describe transport of the ovum from ovary to uterus.
3. Describe transport of sperm from vagina to oviduct.
4. Describe the entry of the sperm into the ovum.
5. Describe the early development of the fertilized ovum, its implantation, and the process of placentation, including descriptions of the blastocyst, trophoblast, and placenta.
6. Describe the hormonal changes during pregnancy; explain why they occur.
7. Define *chorionic gonadotropin,* its chemical nature, site of synthesis, stimuli for release, effector organs, and effect.
8. Describe the basis of the CG pregnancy test.
9. Describe parturition and the accompanying hormonal changes.
10. Predict the effects on uterine motility of increased secretion of progesterone, increased release of oxytocin, and injection of prostaglandins.
11. Describe the glandular structure of the breasts and the hormonal influences that act upon them.
12. Describe the milk letdown reflex; identify the stimuli, receptors, afferent and efferent pathways, integrating center, effector organs, and reflex response.
13. Describe the state of the pituitary gonadotropins during lactation.

Reading Assignment

Chap. 14, pp. 449–458.

Exercises

Directions: Answer the following questions in the space provided.

Oops! Some of the old tried-and-true methods of contraception failed for Ann and Andrew. On Fig. W-71, a diagram of Ann's internal sexual organs, show (using arrows) the routes of sperm and ovum movement, the average times for movement, the normal site of fertilization, and the normal site for implantation of the blastocyst (developing embryo). (*449–450*)

An uneventful nine months come and go and Ann is still carrying her baby. Apparently her body failed to trigger an increased release of oxytocin which would have caused

(*456*)

Her obstetrician decides that an injection of prostaglandins is in order. Ann is injected. What happens? ______________________________ (*456*)

Ann, Jr., is born a normal and healthy child and Ann, Sr., decides she will nurse the baby. Her obstetrician gives her some light bedside reading on the development of mammary glands and lactation so she will completely understand what is happening in her body. The

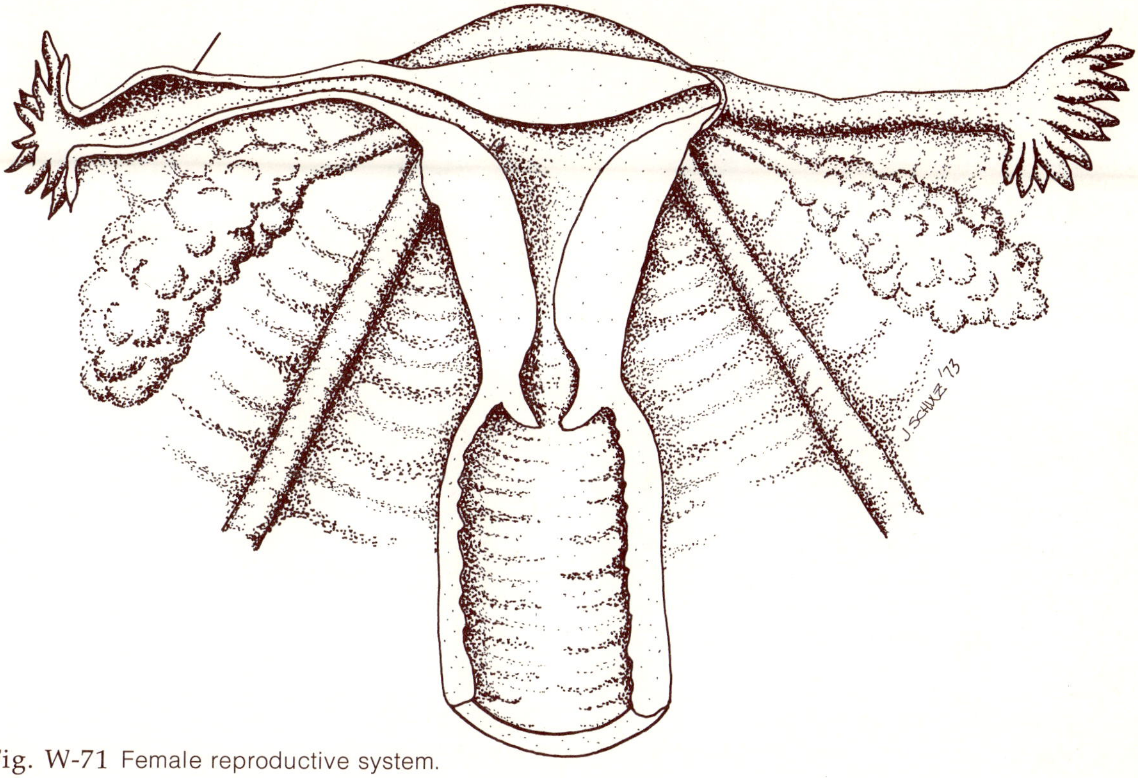

Fig. W-71 Female reproductive system.

accompanying chart appears as a summary in the back of her book. Complete the chart below for Ann. *(456–457)*

Hormone	Effect on Mammary Development and Lactation
1. oxytocin	1. ______________________
2. prolactin-inhibiting factor	2. ______________________
3. progesterone	3. ______________________
4. prolactin	4. ______________________
5. estrogen	5. ______________________
6. growth hormone	6. ______________________

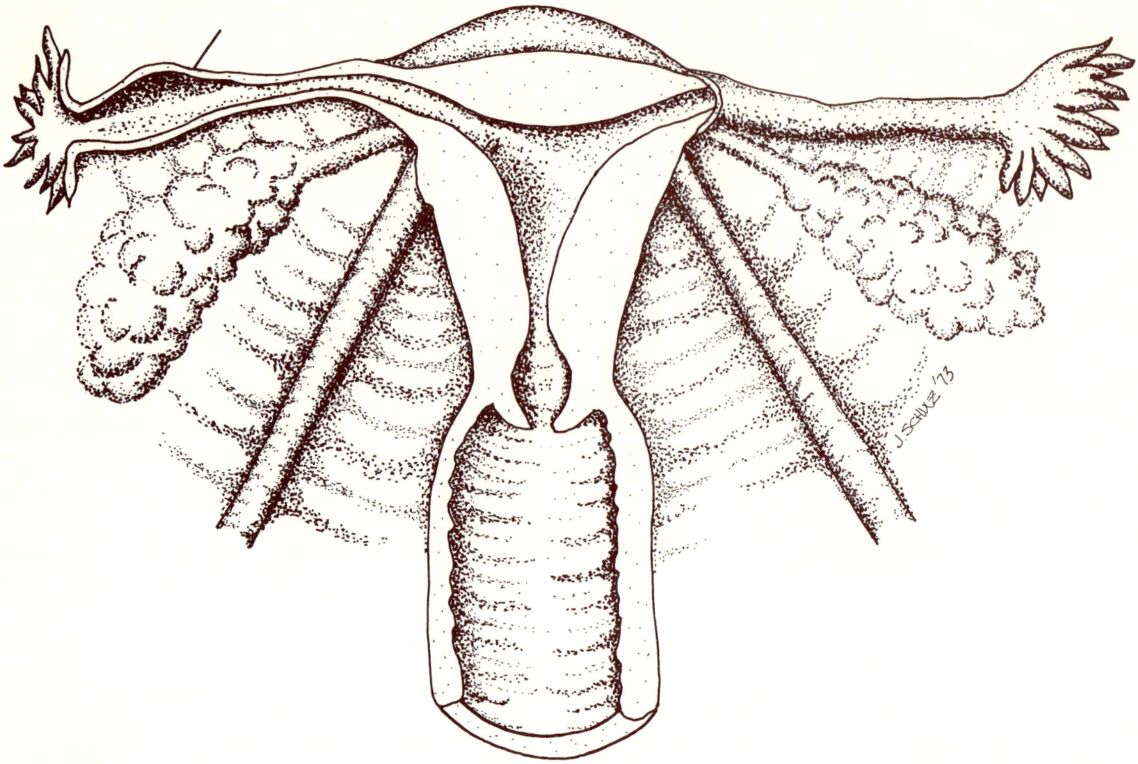

Fig. W-72

Self-Test

Part I

Directions: Using Fig. W-72, a diagram of the female reproductive tract, indicate with arrows

1. the routes of sperm and ovum movement and the average time of movement as follows:
   a sperm—from vagina to site of fertilization.
   b ovum—from release to site of fertilization.
   c ovum—from site of fertilization to site of implantation.
2. a normal site of fertilization.
3. a normal site for implantation.

Part II

Directions: On Fig. W-73, a time diagram for pregnancy, use arrows (⟵⟶) and marks (X) to indicate when each of the listed events occurs. The event of fertilization has been given as an example. Use a separate arrowed line (labeled with the appropriate letter from the list below) for each event.

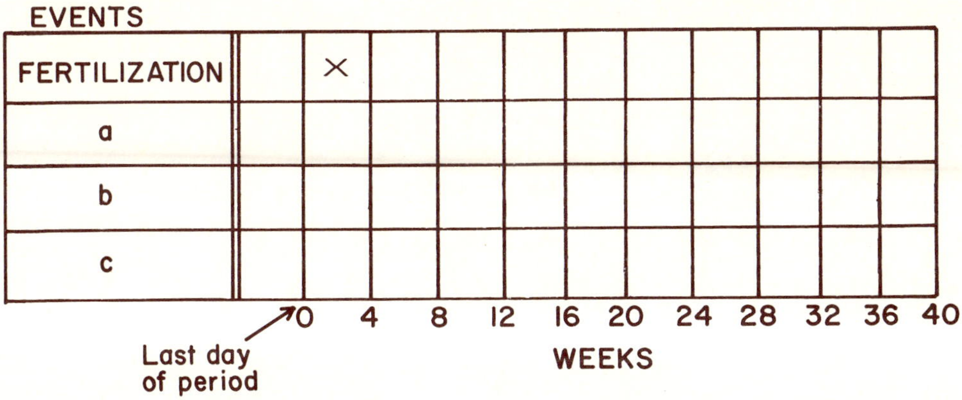

Fig. W-73

Events

a the point at which implantation occurs
b the period during which secretion of the chorionic gonadotropin (CG) occurs
c the period during which the placenta is maintaining pregnancy.

Part III

Directions: In column A on the left below are listed the various hormones acting in mammary development and lactation. In the blank preceding each hormone, write the letter of the function the hormone serves from column B. The items in column B may be used once, more than once, or not at all.

Column A

1. ________ prolactin-inhibiting factor
2. ________ progesterone
3. ________ prolactin
4. ________ estrogen
5. ________ growth hormone
6. ________ oxytocin

Column B

a In large concentration, inhibits milk production
b Controls milk letdown
c Stimulated by testosterone
d Mechanoreceptors in the nipples lead to decreased release
e Stops pregnancy from coming to term
f Stimulates milk secretion
g Secreted by anterior pituitary; necessary for normal breast development
h Ovarian hormone, necessary for breast development

Part IV

Directions: Circle T for true and F for false.

T F 1. Once a sperm is inside an ovum, the zona pellucida's chemical constitution is altered such that it is now impenetrable to other sperm.
T F 2. About 24 hours after fertilization, the blastocyst begins to implant in the uterus.
T F 3. Since CG has LH-like activity, blood or urine from a pregnant woman induces follicular development in female mice or rabbits.

Module IV: Birth Control, Sex Determination, Puberty, and Menopause

Objectives

Upon completion of this module, the student will be able to:

1. Describe the primary means of preventing fertility in men (three) and women (five) (see Table 14-2, p. 459).
2. Select, from a group of curves for cyclical changes in LH release, which one is representative of each of the following situations: a woman on the pill; a normal, untreated woman; a woman with an IUD; and a normal male. (See Exercises.)
3. Contrast sex determination with sex differentiation.
4. Explain what is meant by sexual differentiation of the central nervous system.
5. Define *puberty;* describe the hormonal events involved in it.
6. Describe the physical and hormonal changes during menopause.
7. Describe the sexual changes in males in aging.
8. Differentiate between impotence and sterility.

Reading Assignment

Chap. 14, pp. 458–467.

Supplementary Material

A tubal ligation is becoming an increasingly popular form of birth control. This involves cutting (or cauterizing) the oviducts, preventing the ovum from coming into contact with the sperm. As in a vasectomy, in which the vas deferens is ligated and cut through a small incision made in the scrotal sac (see p. 431), these procedures do not affect the synthesis or release of the reproductive hormones.

Exercises

Part I

Directions: Answer the following questions in the space provided.

1. After several months without using some form of birth control device, Ann is fitted with an IUD. After a month on the IUD, her LH pattern probably looks like which one of the curves in Fig. W-76? ________________________________ *(458–460)*

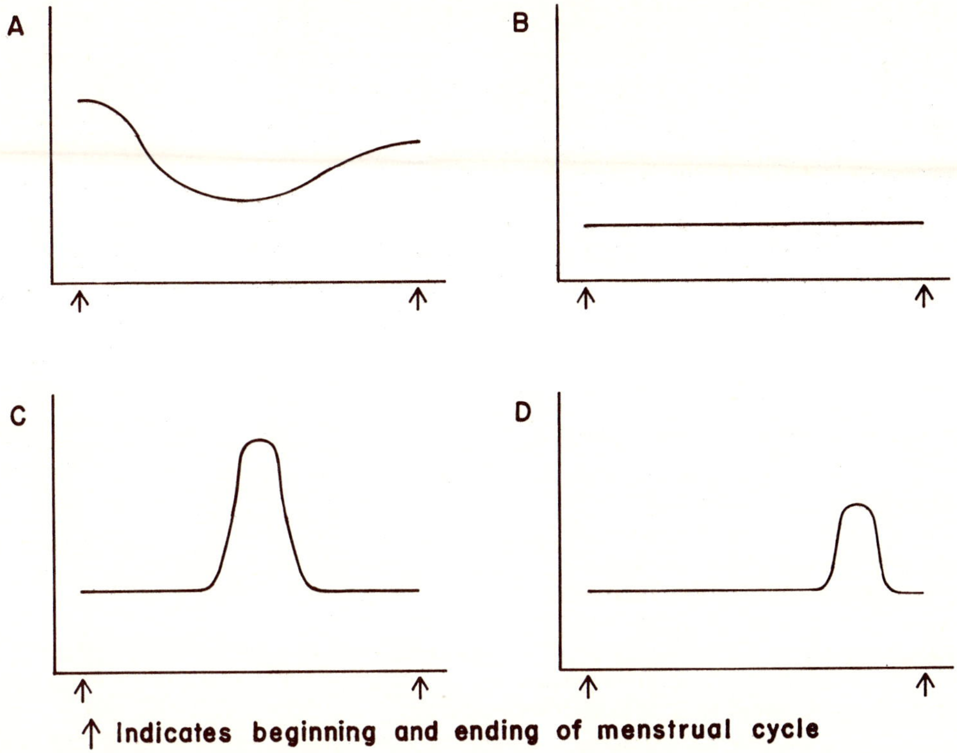

Fig. W-76 LH secretion chart.

2. Ann turns out to be one of those people who has cramps while using an IUD and she returns to her doctor for the pill containing estrogen and progesterone. After a few months on the pill, her LH pattern probably looks like which one of the curves on the chart above?

   ______________________ (458–460)

3. Which of the curves represents Andrew's pattern of LH release?

   ______________________ (438)

Part II

Directions: Answer the following questions in the space provided.

1. Ann begins thinking of having a tubal ligation. What effect will this have on

   a FSH secretion? ______________________

   ______________________ (*Suppl.*)

   b Ann's libido? ______________________

   ______________________ (448)

2. What effect would an ovariectomy have on

   a FSH secretion? ______________________________

   ____

   b Ann's libido? ______________________________

   ______________________________ (448)

Part III

Directions: Answer the following questions in the space provided.

1. Describe the differences between the estrogen and gonadotropin secretion of Ann and that of her mother, who has gone through menopause.

(466–467)

2. What are the physical changes that result from menopause?

Self-Test

Part I

Directions: Use Fig. W-77 to help in answering the following questions. Circle the correct answer(s).

1. Curve A in Fig. W-77 represents LH secretion most typical of

   a a woman on the pill. *b* a castrated male.
   c a woman with an IUD. *d* a normal, untreated woman.

2. Curve B in Fig. W-77 represents an LH secretion most typical of

   a a woman with an IUD. *b* a woman on the pill.
   c a normal, untreated woman. *d* a castrated male.

3. In a woman who has just undergone an ovariectomy but is not taking supplemental hormones,

   a FSH secretion will be increased.
   b FSH secretion will be inhibited.
   c LH secretion will remain unaffected.
   d ovulation will occur regularly.
   e sex drive will be unaffected.

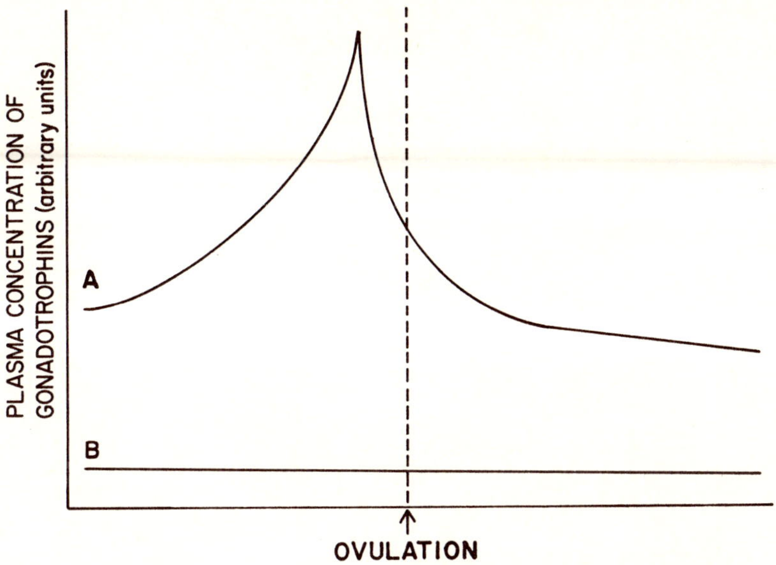

Fig. W-77

Part II

Directions: Answer the following questions in the space provided.

1. Puberty involves an increase in testosterone secretion in the male and an increase in estrogen secretion in the female. What causes release of increased amounts of these hormones?

2. State whether prenatal exposure to estrogen or testosterone is more important in early sexual development.

3. Describe the changes in androgen and gonadotropin secretion in males, with age.

Part III

Directions: Circle T for true and F for false.

T F 1. A tubal ligation involves removal of a small section of the vas deferens.

T F 2. The presence or absence of functioning testes determines development of male or female organs and ducts.

T F 3. A woman with an IUD does not show the normal LH surge which leads to ovulation.

T F 4. One of the effects of menopause is a decrease in protein anabolism resulting in the thinning of the skin and bones.

T F 5. Impotence is the direct result of sterility.

CHAPTER 15 DEFENSE MECHANISMS OF THE BODY

Module I: **Hemostasis**

Objectives

Upon completion of this module, the student will be able to:

1. State the basic prerequisites for bleeding.
2. State why venous bleeding is less serious than arterial bleeding.
3. Define and describe *platelets*.
4. Describe the four hemostatic events prior to clot formation.
5. Diagram the cascade theory of blood clotting as given in Figs. 15-4 and 15-5, p. 473.
6. Describe the roles played by the liver in the overall functioning of the clotting mechanism.
7. Contrast the extrinsic with the intrinsic clotting pathways.
8. Describe clot retraction.
9. Define *serum;* compare serum with plasma.
10. Describe the various roles of platelets in hemostasis (see Fig. 15-7, p. 475).
11. Diagram the anticlotting system and describe its adaptive value.
12. Describe the dominant theories of thrombus formation.
13. Define *thrombosis* and *emboli*.

Reading Assignment

Chap. 15, pp. 468–476.

Exercises

Part I

Directions: Label Fig. W-78 (p. 204) to show the four hemostatic events prior to clot formation (see Fig. 15-2, p. 471, for help).

Part II

Directions: Diagram the role of the liver and vitamin K in the synthesis of plasma clotting factors, prothrombin, and fibrinogen. (See Fig. 15-6, p. 474, to check your answers.)

Part III

Directions: Diagram the cascade theory of blood clotting (see Fig. 15-4, p. 473).

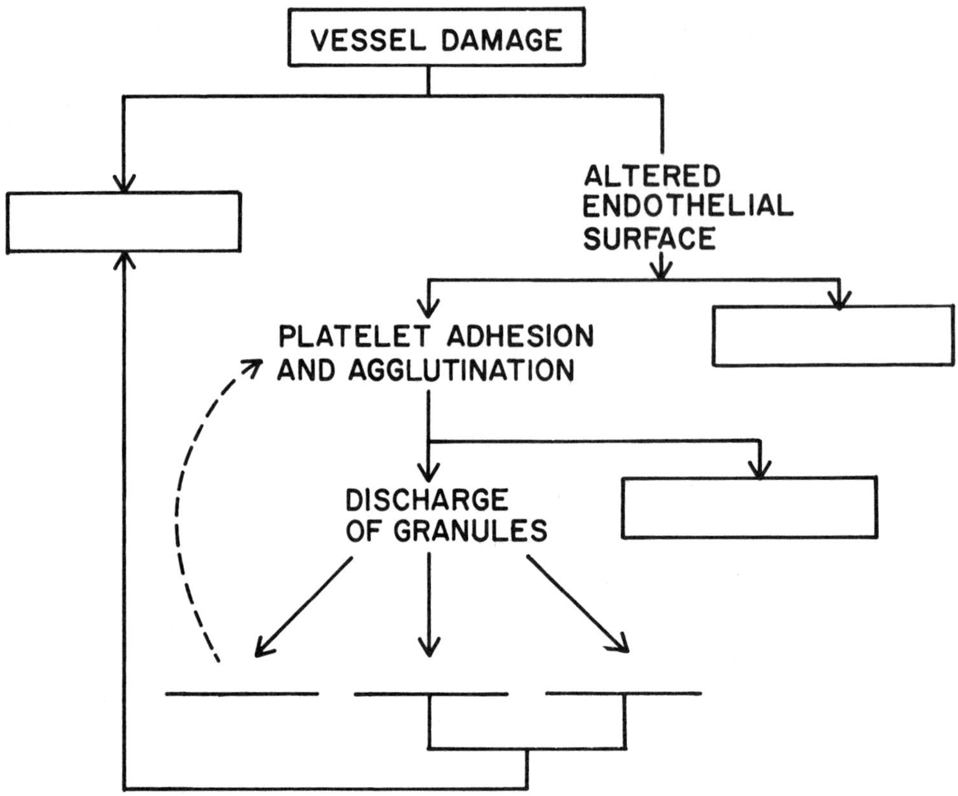

Fig. W-78

Self-Test

Part I

Directions: Complete the following items in the space provided.

1. The basic prerequisites for bleeding are ____

 ____

2. When blood clots, the plasma protein fibrinogen is converted to the fibrous protein fibrin under the influence of an enzyme called ____________________.
3. Platelets originate from certain large cells called

 ____________________.

4. The two vasoconstrictors released from the aggregated platelets which function to maintain vasoconstriction in a small vessel are called

 ____________________ and

 ____________________.

Part II

Directions: Circle T for true and F for false.

T F 1. Individual platelets form clumps and stick to most surfaces as soon as blood is removed for study.

T F 2. The squeezing out of the serum by the pseudopods originating from the mass of agglutinated platelets is called clot retraction.

T F 3. Two naturally occurring anticoagulants are plasmin and thrombin.

Part III

Directions: Answer the following questions in the space provided.

1. Why is venous bleeding less dangerous than arterial bleeding?

2. What is the role of tissue factors in blood clotting?

3. Briefly define

   a platelets ______________________

   b serum ______________________

   c thrombosis ______________________

   d emboli ______________________

Module II: **Immunology, Part I**

Objectives

Upon completion of this module, the student will be able to:

1. Define *immunity* and *immune surveillance.*
2. Describe the specific and nonspecific immune responses.
3. State the two categories of specific immunity and their mediators.
4. List four ways in which bacteria or viruses harm man.

5. List the major effector cells of the immune system.
6. Define a *leukocyte,* and state where leukocytes perform their function.
7. Describe the granulocytes and state their functions.
8. Define *monocyte* and *macrophage,* and state the relation between them.
9. Define *lymphocyte,* and state its function.

Reading Assignment

Chap. 15, pp. 476–480.

Exercises

Part I

Directions: Answer the following questions in the space provided.

1. List the five different types of effector cells of the immune system. *(477)*

   a ____________ *b* ____________

   c ____________ *d* ____________

   e ____________

2. Name and describe the three types of granulocytes. *(477–478)*

   a ____________

   b ____________

   c ____________

Part II

Distinguish between immunity and immune surveillance. *(476)*

Part III

Directions: Many of the effector cells of the immune system are found within the lymphoid tissues. On Fig. W-79, label the locations of the lymphoid tissue. What lymphoid areas are not labeled? (See Fig. 15-10, p. 478, for answers.)

Self-Test

Part I

Directions: Complete the following items in the space provided.

1. Immune responses may be classified into what two categories?

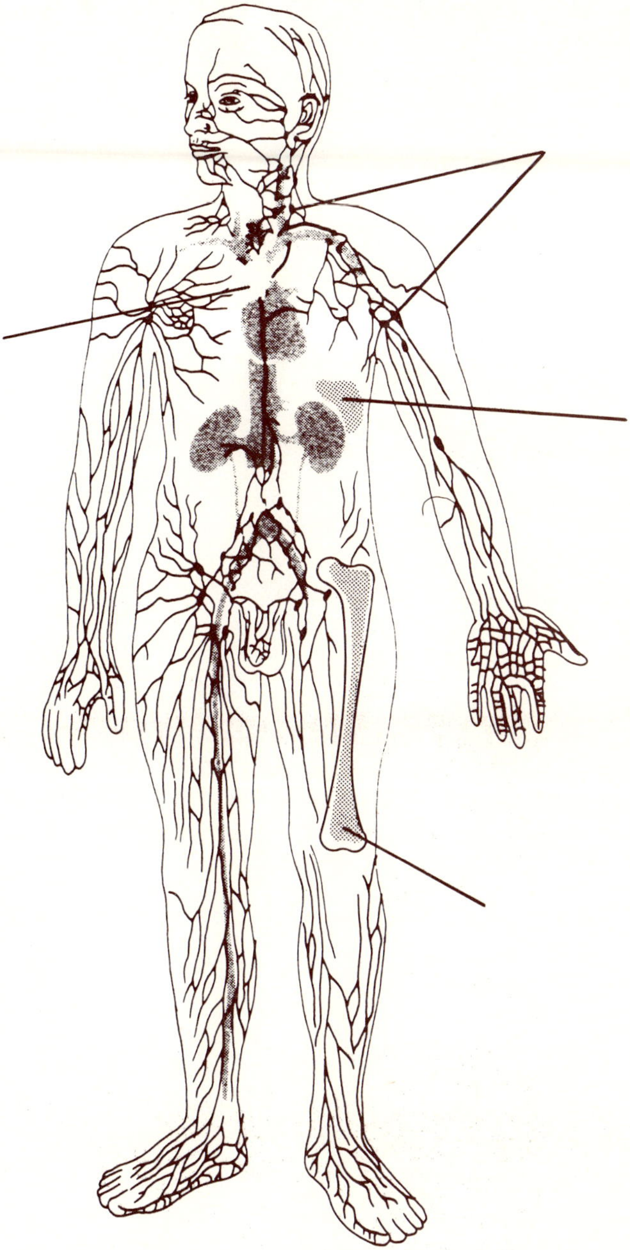

Fig. W-79

a ______________________________

b ______________________________

2. Humoral and cell-mediated immunity are the function of

______________________ cells.

3. Humoral immunity is mediated by circulating ________________

and cell-mediated immunity is mediated by ________________.
4. The five major effector cells of the immune systems are:

a ________________ *b* ________________

c ________________ *d* ________________

e ________________

5. The neutrophils, eosinophils, and basophils are produced in the

________________.
6. Four ways in which microorganisms cause damage and endanger health are

a ________________

b ________________

c ________________

d ________________

Part II

Directions: Circle T for true and F for false.

T F 1. Specific immune responses are dependent upon prior exposure to the foreign substance.

T F 2. The nonspecific defense mechanisms rely on the lymphoid cells for humoral and cell-mediated immune responses.

T F 3. The major functions of leukocytes are exerted within the blood vessels.

Part III

Directions: Complete the following items in the space provided.

1. What is the difference between humoral and cell-mediated immunity?

2. Define briefly:

a immunity

b monocytes

c lymphocytes

Module III: Immunology, Part II

Objectives

Upon completion of this module, the student will be able to:

1. List the external anatomic and chemical defenses against infection.
2. List the sequence of events in a local infection.
3. List the chemical mediators of the vascular changes to nonspecific inflammatory responses as histamine and the kinins.
4. Describe the pathways for histamine release (see Fig. 15-12).
5. Describe the pathways for kinin generation (see Fig. 15-13).
6. Describe the positive-feedback relation between plasma kininogen and tissue kallikrein.
7. Define *neutrophil exudation* and *chemotaxis.*
8. State the positive-feedback relation between kinin and the neutrophils.
9. Describe phagocytosis; list the phagocytic cell types (see also p. 478).
10. Describe abscess and granuloma formation.
11. State the relation between inflammation and fever.
12. Define and describe the *function of interferon.*

Reading Assignment

Chap. 15, pp. 480–486.

Exercises

Part I

Directions: In the space below, draw a diagram to show the pathways for kinin generation in the nonspecific inflammatory reactions once the microbes have entered the body, and showing also the role of activated Hageman factor in the whole process. (See Fig. 15-13, p. 481, to check your answers.)

Part II

Directions: In the space below, draw a diagram to show the pathways for histamine release in nonspecific inflammatory reactions once the microbes have entered the body. (See Fig. 15-12, p. 481, to check your answers.)

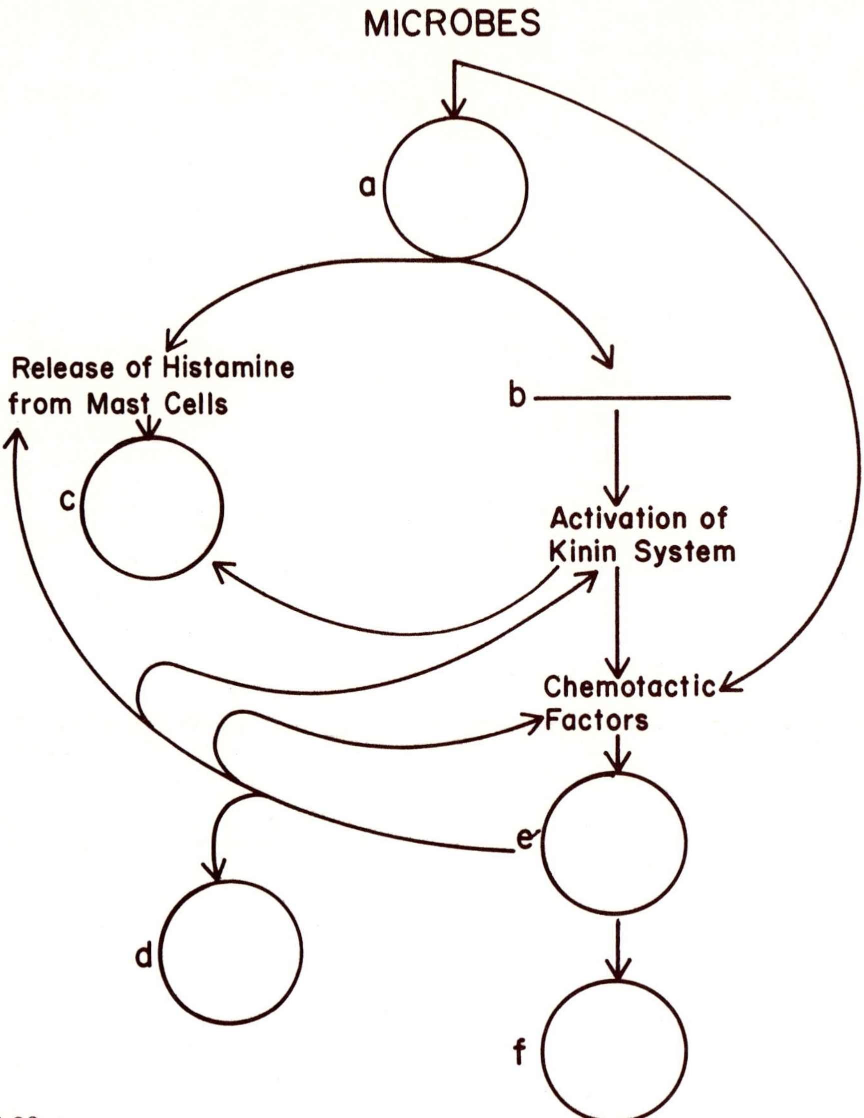

Fig. W-80

Part III

Directions: Complete Fig. W-80 to show a summary of the nonspecific local inflammatory response to infection. (See Fig. 15-18, p. 487, for help.)

Self-Test

Part I

Directions: Complete the following items in the space provided.

1. Number (1 through 7) the following sequence of events in a local infection:

a ________ exit of neutrophils (and later monocytes) from the vessels into the tissues

b ________ repair of tissue

c ________ initial entry of microbes

d ________ phagocytosis and destruction of the microbes

e ________ filtration of fluid into the tissue with resultant swelling

f ________ vasodilation of all vessels of the microcirculation leading to increased blood flow

g ________ a marked increase in vascular permeability to protein

2. The biological function of inflammation is ________________________________.
3. The major direct chemical mediators of vascular changes in nonspecific inflammatory responses are ________________________________ and ________________________________.
4. Within 30 to 60 min after the onset of inflammation an interaction occurs between the vascular endothelium and the circulatory neutrophils, resulting in ________________________________.
5. Histamine is particularly concentrated in what three cell types?

   a ________________________________

   b ________________________________

   c ________________________________

Part II

Directions: Circle T for true and F for false.

T F 1. Hageman factor is, itself, inactive until activated locally, by contact with altered vascular surface.

T F 2. Active kallikrein is only found in neutrophils.

T F 3. In the nonspecific inflammatory response, regeneration of organ-specific cells occurs in muscle and in the central nervous system.

Part III

Directions: Complete the following items in the space provided.

1. What is the relationship between inflammation and fever?

   ____

2. What is the primary function of the nonspecific inflammatory response? ________________

   ____

3. What is leukocytosis?

4. Define briefly:
   a chemotaxis ______________________________
   b interferon ______________________________
   c abscess ______________________________
   d granuloma ______________________________

Module IV: Immunology, Part III

Objectives

Upon completion of this module, the student will be able to:

1. Name and state the functions of the two cell populations involved in the specific immune system.
2. Define *antibody* and *antigen.*
3. Describe antibody specificity and its structural basis.
4. State the major function of antigen-antibody complexes.
5. Define *complement;* list the functions of activated complement proteins as depicted in Fig. 15-22, p. 490.
6. Describe the direct neutralization of bacterial toxins and viruses by antibodies.
7. Describe the production of antibodies.
8. Contrast active with passive immunity.
9. Describe the mechanisms of cell-mediated immunity.
10. Describe the interplay between nonspecific and specific immune mechanisms in resisting infection.
11. List the factors which alter resistance to infection.
12. Describe the way cancer cells are normally destroyed.
13. Describe immune enhancement.

Reading Assignment

Chap. 15, pp. 486–496.

Exercises

Directions: Answer the following questions in the space provided.

1. You have a relative who has leukemia and who may have tremendous numbers of blood neutrophils or monocytes (note that infection increases the number of leukocytes). Why might this leukemia patient be extremely prone to infection? *(495)*

2. You have a patient who has skin cancer. What kind of immunity is capable of recognizing and destroying cancer cells? What feature of these cells causes them to be recognized as "foreign"? *(495–496)*

3. Briefly outline the functions of complement (see Fig. 15-22, p. 490). How do certain of these actions aid the nonspecific inflammatory response (as illustrated in Fig. 15-18, p. 487)?

Self-Test

Part I

Directions: Circle T for true and F for false.

T F 1. T cells enter the thymus after their release from the bone marrow.
T F 2. The B cells, responsible for humoral immune responses, differentiate into antibody-producing cells.
T F 3. The body normally secretes large amounts of cortisol when a person is under psychic or physical stress.
T F 4. All microorganisms induce active immunity.
T F 5. B cells are the major carriers of specific immunity against fungi, viruses, and parasites.
T F 6. Macrophages play a crucial role in antibody synthesis.

Part II

Directions: Complete the following items in the space provided.

1. Antibodies all belong to the family of proteins known as

   ______________________ or ______________________.

2. ______________________ acts as an amplification system for inflammation in humoral immunity.
3. The activators of the initial step in the complement sequence are ______________________

   ______________________.

Part III

Directions: Complete the following items in the space provided.

1. When B lymphocytes are stimulated, they undergo cell division which produces

   ______________________ cells, the active

   ______________________ producers.

2. How do antibodies neutralize bacterial toxins?

3. Antibiotics work by ____.
4. What is the difference between active and passive immunity?

5. Differentiate between an antibody and its antigen.

Module V: Immunology, Part IV

Objectives

Upon completion of this module, the student will be able to:

1. Define *histocompatibility antigen.*
2. Describe the mechanisms of tissue rejection.
3. List three methods of combatting rejection.
4. Explain the relation between tissue rejection and transfusion reactions; state the differences between them.
5. Predict what will happen if a type A person is given type B blood.
6. Describe the Rh antibody-antigen system.
7. Define the equivalent terms, *allergy* and *hypersensitivity.*
8. Distinguish between atopic allergy and autoimmune disease.
9. Describe the mechanism of the atopic allergic response.
10. List five of the causes for the body's failure to recognize its own cells.

Reading Assignment

Chap. 15, pp. 496–499.

Exercises

Directions: Answer the following questions in the space provided.

1. If a type A person is given type B blood, the anti-A antibody in the transfused plasma causes the recipient's cells to be attacked. How serious is this consequence and why? (497)

2. You have a patient whose blood type is AB. What type(s) of blood can this patient receive and why? *(497)*

3. Type O people are frequently called universal blood donors. What makes this statement correct? *(497)*

4. You have a patient who has been treated by radiation and drugs to reduce tissue rejection. How do these two treatments act to reduce tissue rejection? What might be the undesirable side effect(s) of using radiation and drugs? *(496)*

5. Describe the causes of the allergic reaction of a hayfever sufferer. *(498)*

6. How does desensitization help to block the inflammatory response? *(499)*

Self-Test

Part I

Directions: Circle the correct answer(s).

1. An acquired reactivity to an antigen which can result in bodily damage upon subsequent exposure to that particular antigen is called

   a allergy. *b* histocompatibility.
   c hypersensitivity. *d* interferon.

2. The use of radiation and drugs to reduce tissue rejection results in

   a decrease in T cells.
   b increase in B cells.
   c decrease in B cells.
   d increase in actively dividing lymphocytes.

3. People with type O blood can receive

   a A. *b* B. *c* AB. *d* O.

Part II

Directions: Circle T for true and F for false.

T F 1. Type O people are frequently called universal donors and type AB people are universal recipients.

T F 2. Everybody is born with anti-Rh antibodies.

T F 3. When tissue is transplanted from one person to another, the transplanted cells are destroyed by circulating B cells.

T F 4. An autoimmune damage may occur by excess generation of complement or release of chemicals from platelets, neutrophils, or sensitized lymphocytes in response to invading foreign cells.

T F 5. Graft recipients receiving medication to reduce their T cell activity manifest an increased tendency to develop certain types of cancer.

Part III

Directions: Answer the following questions in the space provided.

1. What are the three most important erythrocyte membrane antigens?

   ____

2. What are the two incompatibilities that arise when a type A person is given type B blood?

   a

   b

3. List five reasons that the body can fail to recognize its own cells (autoimmune disease).

   a ____________________________________

   b ____________________________________

   c ____________________________________

   d ____________________________________

   e ____________________________________

Module VI: **Resistance to Stress**

Objectives

Upon completion of this module, the student will be able to:

1. State the responses common to almost all types of stress.
2. List cortisol's effects on organic metabolism and state their adaptive value.

3. State the relation between the sympathetic nervous system and cortisol in stress.
4. List the pharmacological effects of cortisol.
5. List the eight major effects of increased sympathetic activity during stress.
6. List the other hormones that are released during stress and state their adaptive value.

Reading Assignment

Chap. 15, pp. 499–502.

Exercises

Directions: Complete the following items in the space provided.

1. Identify the effects cortisol has on the following. *(500)*

   a protein catabolism ____________________

   b liver uptake of amino acids ____________________

   c glucose uptake and oxidation ____________________

   d stimulation of gluconeogenesis ____________________

2. Suppose you have a patient who is lacking cortisol and who is faced with a moderate stress. What might be the effect of that on his health and why? *(500–501)*

3. Indicate whether cortisol secretion increases, decreases, or remains the same in each of the following situations. *(501)*

   a awaiting surgical operation ____________________

   b during final exams ____________________

   c during job interview ____________________

Self-Test

Part I

Directions: Complete the following items in the space provided.

1. The two responses common to most types of stress are:

   a ____________________

   b ____________________

2. When cortisol is present in very high concentration, there may appear new effects known as ____________________.
3. Briefly describe the pathway for increased cortisol secretion.

Part II

Directions: Circle the correct answer(s).

1. Normal cardiovascular response to stress requires

   a increased cortisol secretion.
   b decreased cortisol secretion.
   c no change in cortisol secretion.

2. Large amounts of cortisol may result in

   a an increase in antibody production.
   b a decrease in antibody production.
   c inhibition of phagocytosis.
   d inhibition of vasodilation.

3. A diabetic who suffers an infection requires

   a much more insulin than usual.
   b much less insulin than usual.
   c no change in insulin.

Part III

Directions: Circle T for true and F for false.

T F 1. Cortisol inhibits glucose uptake and oxidation by the brain.
T F 2. Aldosterone, antidiuretic, and growth hormones are hormones released during different kinds of stress.
T F 3. Certain types of stress can stimulate the sympathetic nervous system without the participation of the hypothalamus.

Part IV

Directions: Circle the number preceding each of the following which are functions of the sympathetic nervous system during stress.

1. increased rate of breathing
2. decreased glycogenolysis
3. increased CNS arousal and alertness
4. redistribution of blood from gastrointestinal tract, kidneys, etc., to skeletal muscle
5. increased blood coagulation
6. increased adipose tissue catabolism
7. increased skeletal muscle fatigue
8. increased cardiac output

Module I:
Basic Characteristics of Sensory Coding

Module II:
Specific Sensory Systems, Part I

Module III:
Specific Sensory Systems, Part II

Module IV:
Levels of Perception

PROCESSING SENSORY INFORMATION

CHAPTER 16

Module I: Basic Characteristics of Sensory Coding

Objectives

Upon completion of this module, the student will be able to:

1. Differentiate between afferent and sensory information.
2. Define *sensory modality* and give several examples of it.
3. Define *sensory unit* and distinguish it from a receptive field.
4. Differentiate between specific and nonspecific ascending pathways.
5. Describe stimulus quality and differentiate between coding of quality and quantity.
6. Differentiate between the somatosensory cortex and the receptive areas for taste, hearing, and sight.
7. Differentiate between the mechanisms for coding in stimulus localization.

Reading Assignment

Chap. 16, pp. 503–509.

Exercises

Directions: Answer the questions in the space provided.

1. Describe the difference between specific and nonspecific sensory ascending neural pathways. *(504)*

2. Name the two mechanisms for coding information on stimulus intensity. *(506)*

3. Primary sensory areas exist in the cerebral cortex. Stimulus (quality/quantity) ________________________________ is indicated by the specific sensitivity of individual receptors conveying information to these areas. *(505)*

4. Which sensory modalities are represented in the somatosensory cortex of the brain? *(505)*

5. What is the variability of threshold potential from the center to the periphery of the receptive field of a single neuron? *(507)*

6. Why are we less able to pinpoint visceral pain (in terms of location) than we are surface or somatic pain? Explain in terms of anatomical differences. *(508)*

7. Diagram in graph form "action potential frequency" (in terms of inhibition and excitation), versus "distance from point of stimulus" to demonstrate the phenomenon of lateral inhibition. (See Fig. 16-7, p. 508, to check your answer.)

Self-Test

Part I

Directions: Circle the correct answer(s).

1. Which of the following describe lateral inhibition?
   a occurs within the receptive field of a single afferent neuron
   b refines and clarifies information about stimulus localization
   c lessens weaker responses and collects stronger ones into a common pathway (intensity contrasts)
   d afferent neurons and interneurons themselves inhibit other parallel afferent components
   e afferent neurons and interneurons inhibit adjacent descending motor neurons

2. The following items relate to stimulus location (L) and/or stimulus intensity (I). Place an L or an I, or both L and I, in the space to the left of each item to indicate your choice of relationship.
   a ________ Threshold stimulus varies in the receptive field.
   b ________ More or fewer sensory units may be activated.

c ________ Frequency of firing of action potential of a sensory unit.

d ________ Specific pathways channel afferent information in a relatively unmixed manner.

e ________ The number, size, and overlap of sensory units affects this parameter.

f ________ Specific afferent pathways carry exclusive information about restricted areas.

3. Which of the following best describe(s) a specific pathway?

   a a single neuron and all the receptor units which innervate it
   b parallel chains of interneurons which are grouped together
   c one which indicates only that something is happening, not what or where
   d afferent neurons and interneurons themselves inhibit other parallel afferent components
   e several sensory units converge upon a given chain of neurons which respond to the same stimulus energy
   f a chain of three to five synaptically connected neuronal links

Part II

Directions: Complete the following items in the space provided.

1. A single afferent neuron plus all the receptor units it innervates make up a

   ______________________________ (2 words).
2. That area which, if stimulated, leads to activity of a neuron is called its

   ______________________________ (2 words).
3. The term applied to the process in which afferent neurons and interneurons themselves

   inhibit other parallel afferent components is ______________________________.
4. Ascending neuronal pathways which are activated by sensory units of several different modalities and therefore convey only general information about the level of excitability

   are termed (specific/nonspecific) pathways. ______________________________
5. A stimulus (quantity/quality) mechanism can be described in terms of sensory units activated and the frequency at which the sensory unit fires.

   ______________________________.

Part III

Directions: Circle T for true and F for false.

T F 1. Stimulus quantity is related to indications by the specific sensitivity of individual receptors and the pathways conveying the information to the primary sensory areas of the brain.

T F 2. All afferent information coming to the central nervous system is called sensory information.

T F 3. The somatosensory cortex of the brain contains fibers subserving the sensory modalities of touch, temperature, taste, sight, and hearing.

T F 4. The placement of a stimulus determines not only the rate at which a single afferent nerve fiber fires, but also the balance of activity within a group of sensory units.

T F 5. Because there is no gradient of sensitivity across the receptive field, the information content of the pattern of activity in a population of afferent neurons is negligible.

T F 6. The precision with which a stimulus can be localized and differentiated from an adjacent stimulus depends on the size of the receptive field conveyed by a single afferent neuron and the amount of overlap of nearby receptive fields.

Module II: Specific Sensory Systems, Part I

Objectives

Upon completion of this module, the student will be able to:

1. Describe the receptor mechanisms for monitoring touch-pressure, joint position, temperature, and pain.
2. Describe in general terms that part of the electromagnetic spectrum that is known to affect the eye.
3. Describe accommodation and its role in focusing an image on the retina.
4. Define *myopic* vision, *hyperopic* vision, and *astigmatism,* and the defect responsible for each.
5. Differentiate between the function of rods and cones and describe their role in visual acuity and dark adaptation.
6. List the elements of the visual pathway in order of processing visual information (Fig. 16-19).
7. Describe the relationship between receptive fields and the simple, complex, and hypercomplex cells of the visual cortex.
8. List the four types of eye movements and describe the adaptive value of each.

Reading Assignment

Chap. 16, pp. 509–522.

Exercises

Directions: Answer the following questions in the space provided.

1. What are the four types of specific sensory systems? *(509–510)*

2. Describe how each of the four sensory system receptors functions to send input to the central nervous system. *(509–510)*

3. What is the wavelength portion of the electromagnetic spectrum to which the receptors of the eye are sensitive? (*511*)

4. Why does a blue sky look blue and not green? (Describe in terms of light receptor function.) (*511*)

5. What does the lens of the eye do in the process of accommodation?

    ______________________________ (2 words) (*512*)

6. Accommodation is (easier/more difficult) for older people.

    ______________________________ (*512*)

7. Which of the two types of visual receptor cell is responsible for dark vision, visual acuity, color perception, and brightness? (*514–515*)

8. Show the order of elements of the visual pathway by filling in the spaces in Fig. W-81. (See Fig. 16-19, p. 515.)
9. Using diagrams, show how a stimulus must be applied to produce increased rates of firing of *complex* cortical cells. (See Fig. 16-24, p. 519.)

10. State the configuration of receptive fields to which the simple and the complex cells are sensitive. (*518*)

11. List four types of eye movements and give examples of each. (*521*)

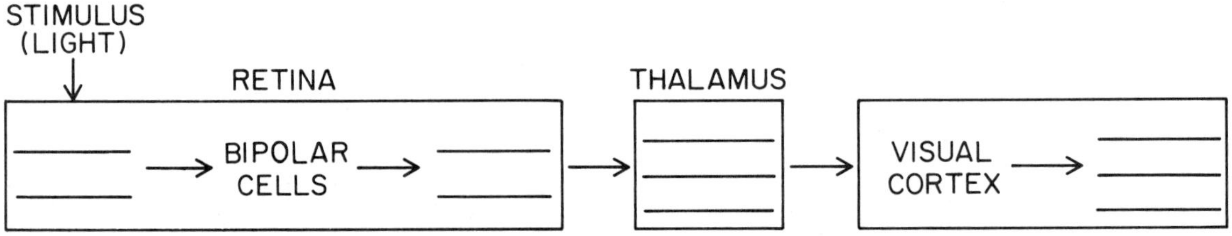

Fig. W-81

Self-Test

Part I

Directions: Circle T for true and F for false.

T F 1. By receptor, we mean the afferent-nerve fiber ending *plus* the specialized nonneural cells associated with it.
T F 2. The pacinian corpuscle signals pressure.
T F 3. All joint receptors fire faster in extension than in flexion.
T F 4. The current theory of the source of a high-temperature signal is via generator potentials caused by changes in protein molecule configuration of the receptor.
T F 5. Hot and cold receptor mechanisms are thought to be the same.
T F 6. The sensation of pain cannot be separated from the emotional and behavioral reaction.
T F 7. The entire electromagnetic spectrum is detected by the eye.
T F 8. The change in shape of the cornea to focus the visual image is called accommodation.
T F 9. Both the cornea and the lens function to focus the visual image on the retina.
T F 10. Visual acuity in dim light is due in part to the shift from rod to cone receptors.
T F 11. The visual system does not form a picture in the brain, but through the simultaneous activation of many neurons it forms a specifically coded electrical statement.
T F 12. Cortical cells of the primary visual cortex may be classified as either simple or complex according to the stimuli to which they respond.

Part II

Directions: Circle the correct answer(s).

1. A pacinian corpuscle is a receptor for which of the following?

   a temperature *b* pain
   c joint position *d* touch pressure changes

2. Receptors signaling joint position are activated by which of the following stimuli?

   a light pressure on the skin of the arm
   b stretching to take a book off a high shelf
   c twisting or rotating the arm as in turning a door knob
   d normal movements such as walking
   e no movement at all
   f painful movements such as those felt by most people trying to touch their wrist with their thumb

3. The stimuli which give rise to pain result in which of the following?

   a sensory experience
   b reaction including emotional and behavioral responses
   c neither of the above

4. Which of the following are true regarding the pain sensory system?

   a two ascending pathways to the brain are probably used simultaneously
   b the pathway to the cerebral cortex arouses the aversive reactive response to the stimulus

c the pathway to the brainstem reticular formation is involved in perception of the pain stimulus
d receptors fire more rapidly as the stimulus severity increases
e the specific pathway ascends to the thalamus and the cerebral cortex
f descending pathways can alter the transmission of information in afferent neurons

5. The wavelengths capable of stimulating the eye receptors are limited to

a 250–700 nm. *b* 400–700 cm.
c 300–600 mm. *d* 540–565 nm.
e none of the given measures

6. Simple cells of the primary visual cortex have receptive fields which are

a concentric on-off, i.e., circular.
b side by side with straight boundaries.
c sensitive only to a moving stimulus.

Part III

Directions: Fill in the blanks as indicated.

1. The process of changing the shape of the lens to adjust for distance in focusing the visual image on the retina is called ____________________________.
2. Match the items in column A with those in column B. Answers may be used more than once.

		Column A	Column B
I	______	Sometimes referred to as a nearsighted eye	*a* farsighted
II	______	Sometimes referred to as a farsighted eye	*b* nearsighted
III	______	Far objects focused in front of the retina	*c* myopic
IV	______	Near objects focused behind the retina	*d* hyperopic
V	______	Irregularities in the cornea	*e* astigmatism
VI	______	Can be corrected or compensated for by eyeglasses	*f* cataract
VII	______	Results when the eyeball is too long for the lens size	*g* accommodation
VIII	______	Results when the eyeball is too short for the lens size	*h* retina

3. The following are statements describing rod and/or cone receptor cells of the eye. Indicate whether the statement describes a rod (R), a cone (C), or both (R, C).

I ______ contain light-sensitive molecules called photopigments

II ______ are most numerous in the peripheral retina

III ______ act as photoreceptors during conditions of poor illumination and for night vision

IV ______ have very high visual acuity

V ______ indicate brightness

VI ________ indicate color

VII ________ synapses on a bipolar cell

4. Arrange the following items in the proper order to show the processing of visual information.

I ________ visual cortex

II ________ Ganglion cells

III ________ stimulus

IV ________ rods and cones

V ________ visual association cortex

VI ________ lateral geniculate nucleus

VII ________ bipolar cells

5. Primary visual cortex cells which have receptive fields that are divided into off and on regions, all having a side-by-side arrangement of excitatory and inhibitory areas with straight boundaries rather than circular ones, are called

____ cells.

6. Primary visual cortex cells which respond to a line in a particular orientation across the receptive field only when the stimulus is in motion across the visual field are called

____ cells.

7. Hypercomplex cells of the primary visual cortex are activated in the visual pathway by

____ cells.

8. What are the four types of eye movement?

a ____

b ____

c ____

d ____

9. Match the following items describing eye-movement control.

	Column A	Column B
I ________	tracks object through depth of visual field	*a* tracking of visual objects
II ________	smooth movements throughout visual field	*b* search for visual targets
III ________	small rapid jerks	*c* adaptation
IV ________	adjusts visual field in opposite direction of head movement	*d* compensation for head movements
		e convergence

Module III: Specific Sensory Systems, Part II

Objectives

Upon completion of this module, the student will be able to:

1. Define *frequency, amplitude,* and *purity* in relation to the reception of sound by the ear.
2. Describe the transmission of sound from the atmosphere to the oval window, including the role of each structure in the outer and middle ear.
3. Describe the role of the oval window, basilar membrane, scala vestibuli, scala tympani, and the hair cells in the reception of sound.
4. Describe the mechanisms for localizing the source of a sound.
5. Describe the basic structural elements of the vestibular system and their role in detection of motion and position.
6. Describe the receptor mechanisms for taste and smell.

Reading Assignment

Chap. 16, pp. 522–532.

Exercises

Directions: Answer the questions in the space provided.

1. Explain why a person could not be heard talking in a perfect vacuum. *(522)*

2. Explain what is meant by a "pure" tone. *(523)*

3. What is the difference between frequency and amplitude of a sound? *(523)*

4. The cells which generate impulses corresponding to sounds coming into the ear are called ________________________________. Describe the mechanism of how they function. *(524–525)*

5. What part of the basilar membrane responds to high-pitch sounds? Low-pitch sounds? *(524)*

6. Why is the force per unit area on the oval window 15 to 20 times greater than that on the tympanic membrane? *(524)*

7. What is wrong with the following sequence of events in the transmission of sound in the ear?

   Ear canal → tympanic membrane → middle ear bones → oval window → scala tympani → scala vestibuli
   scala tympani → basilar membrane → hair cells and tectorial membrane → generator potential *(524)*

8. The two most important clues in finding a sound source are

   ________________________________ and

   ________________________________. *(526)*

9. The two main functions of the vestibular system are to

   ________________________________ and to

   ________________________________. These functions are performed by structures known respectively as the ________________________________ and the

   ____________________ and ____________________ *(526)*

10. The system for sensing taste can differentiate both quality and quantity. Explain how these differ in terms of firing of action potentials of specific taste receptors. *(530–531)*

11. Explain the difference in sensitivity and discrimination capability between taste and smell receptor cells. *(530–532)*

Self-Test

Part I

Directions: Fill in the blanks as indicated.

1. Match the following.

	Column A	Column B
I ________	loudness of a sound	*a* purity
II ________	number of sound frequencies in addition to the fundamental tone	*b* frequency
III ________	related to the pitch of the sound	*c* amplitude
		d timbre

2. Match the structure of the ear with its function.

	Column A	Column B
I ________	transfers movements of the air in the outer ear to the fluid-filled chambers of the inner ear	*a* oval window
II ________	couples the tympanic membrane with the oval window	*b* cochlea
III ________	transmits sound (pressure) waves to the tympanic membrane	*c* ear canal
IV ________	separates the middle and inner ear	*d* middle ear bones
V ________	senses sound waves coming through the ear canal	*e* eustachian tube
		f tympanic membrane

3. Choose the proper sequence of events in the transmission of sound through the middle and inner ear.

I ________ The region of maximal displacement of basilar membrane varies with the frequency of vibration of the sound source.

II ________ Where the displacement of basilar membrane is a maximum, the stimulation of the hair cell receptors which ride on the membrane is the greatest.

III ________ The pressure wave passes up the ear canal and pushes in on the tympanic membrane.

IV ________ A wave of pressure is produced in the scala vestibuli on the inner ear side of the oval window.

V ________ Most of the pressure waves are transmitted to the basilar membrane which is deflected into the scala tympani.

VI ________ The chain of bones rocks the foot plate of the stapes against the oval window causing it to bow into the inner ear.

VII ________ In the normal hearing, the greater potentials formed by the activated cells lead ultimately to the production of action potentials in the peripheral endings of the afferent nerves, the resulting action potentials being transmitted to the central nervous system.

4. The mechanisms most important in localization of a sound source are

5. The vestibular system contains mechanoreceptors specialized to detect changes in

____________________ and

____________________.

6. Match the following:

_____ semicircular canals	*a* rate of change of motion of the head
_____ utricle and saccule	*b* provides information about the position of the head relative to the direction of forces of gravity

Part II

Directions: Circle the correct answer(s).

1. Which of the following are structures of the inner ear?

a stapes
b scala vestibuli
c scala tympani
d eustachian tube
e tectorial membrane
f cochlea
g basilar membrane
h hair cells
i tympanic membrane

2. Which of the following is (are) true for the basilar membrane?

a magnifies the sound impulse
b sorts out incoming sound waves along its length
c supports sound receptors called hair cells
d is associated with a structure called the tectorial membrane
e is more elastic closer to the oval window
f divides the cochlea into the scala vestibuli and the scala tympani

3. Which of the following is (are) true for sound localization?

a A sound on the left stimulates the left ear before it stimulates the right ear.
b Difference in time onset is most useful in localizing low-frequency sounds.
c A difference in intensity is most useful in localizing high-frequency sounds.
d In man the cerebral cortex is necessary for actual sound localization.

4. Which of the following is (are) true of the vestibular apparatus?

a detects direction of sound
b is a membranous sac
c is in the temporal bone of the skull
d contains three semicircular canals
e contains hair cells which vibrate faster with louder sound input
f contains a slight bulge for the utricle and saccule
g contains endolymph

5. Which of the following is (are) correct for taste reception?
   - *a* Quality of taste is transmitted by the frequency of action potentials from receptor cells.
   - *b* Individual molecules of a chemical substance bind with specific sites on the receptor cell membrane.
   - *c* The chemical substance-receptor site combination alters the cell membrane potential.
   - *d* The membrane of the receptor cell depolarizes when the cell is stimulated chemically.
   - *e* Quantity of taste is related to variation of relative sensitivity of receptor cells in a group of neurons.

6. Olfactory *discrimination* depends on which of the following?
   - *a* action potential pattern generated in the different afferent neurons
   - *b* histological appearance of the receptor cell
   - *c* head congestion in the nasal passages
   - *d* physical alertness
   - *e* patency of the eustachian tube
   - *f* hunger
   - *g* sex
   - *h* smoking
   - *i* blood pressure

Part III

Directions: Circle T for true and F for false.

T F 1. The pressure on the tympanic membrane is the same as that on the oval window for the same impulse.

T F 2. Most sound impulses passing through the oval window travel the full length of the scala vestibuli, then pass into the scala tympani.

T F 3. Sound impulses passing from the scala vestibuli into the scala tympani without being transmitted by the basilar membrane are likely to be of low pitch rather than high pitch.

T F 4. Otoliths are tiny calcium carbonate stones found only in the endolymph fluid of the semicircular canals.

T F 5. The hair cells of the semicircular canals are stimulated only during changes in rate of motion.

T F 6. The utricle and saccule contain the receptors of the vestibular system which provide information about the positon of the head relative to the direction of the forces of gravity.

T F 7. Current theory relating to taste sensation states that there are separate and distinct cells for each of the basic taste sensations, and action potentials are fired when a chemical substance related to that basic category contacts the cell.

T F 8. The frequency of action potentials in single nerve fibers increases in response to increasing concentrations of the chemical stimulant.

T F 9. Awareness of a specific taste of a substance probably depends upon the relative activity in a number of different neurons rather than that in a specific neuron.

T F 10. Receptor mechanisms for smell are probably differentiated at the chemical substance-receptor site level.

T F 11. The olfactory cells are differentiated into basic groups for specific odor sensations as are those for taste.

Module IV: **Levels of Perception**

Objectives

Upon completion of this module, the student will be able to:

1. Differentiate between the roles of the somatosensory and cortical association areas of the cortex in the process of perception.
2. List and describe four factors known to distort our perception.
3. Differentiate between perception and sensory input.
4. Differentiate between false information received by a receptor and a perceptual illusion.

Reading Assignment

Chap. 16, pp. 532–536.

Exercises

Part I

Directions: Fill in the blanks as indicated.

1. Match the following:

________ required for higher mental activity	*a* somatosensory cortex	
________ required for basic sensory modality	*b* cortical association area	
________ connects primary cortical sensory or motor areas		
________ elaborates sensory information		*(532–533)*

2. List four factors known to distort our perception.

   a ________________________________

   b ________________________________

   c ________________________________

   d ________________________________ *(533–534)*

3. Match the following:

________ brain's analysis of events	*a* sensory input *b* perception	
________ information obtained at the receptor level		
________ modified by many factors		
________ always a conscious event		
________ has many levels		*(534–536)*

Part II

1. Is there a difference in perception at the cortical level between false information (such as electrical stimulation of a receptor) and a perceptual illusion? Explain. (*534*)

Self-Test

Part I

Directions: Fill in the blanks as indicated.

1. A part of the brain which, when lost, results in the loss of a specific sense (example: sight) is known as ______________________.
2. That part of the brain which is able to add further elaboration to a basic sense and is of great importance in the maintenance of higher mental activities is called a(n) ______________________.
3. Indicate by entering an A or an S whether the statement describes the association cortex (A) or the somatosensory cortex (S).

   I ________ Permits logical interpretation of perceptions.

   II ________ Loss of this part of the brain results in the loss of a specific modality.

   III ________ Allows information processing for appropriateness.

   IV ________ Compares information received by one sensory modality with that of another sensory modality.

   V ________ Is of great importance in maintenance of higher mental activities.

4. Match the following:

   I ________ Contrary to our perceptual learning.

   II ________ Damage to the receptor.

   III ________ Action potentials in a given afferent pathway going to a certain area of the brain signal the kind of information normally carried in the pathway (i.e., stimulus can be in the form of electrical or action potential).

   IV ________ Can be proved false by physical measurements.

   V ________ Occurs at the receptor level.

   VI ________ Occurs at the cortical level, i.e., does not fit previous pattern.

   a false information
   b perceptual illusion

Part II

Directions: Circle T for true and F for false.

T F 1. Sensory input can be learned as part of system development.

T F 2. Perception is a function of system development and learning.

T F 3. Sensory input is that information supplied at the receptor level, while perception is what the brain says is happening after nervous system alteration, combinations, modifications, and omissions have occurred.

T F 4. Sensory input is what happens, while perception is what the brain "sees."

Part III

Directions: Circle the correct answer(s).

1. Which of the following describe factors known to distort our perceptions?

   a afferent information distorted by receptor mechanisms and by its processing along afferent pathways

   b events experienced the very first time

   c loss of the somatosensory cortex

   d emotions, personality, and social background

   e lack of suitable receptors for many energy forms

   f information entering the central nervous system but not giving rise to conscious sensations

Module I:
Local Control of Motor Neurons

Module II:
Descending Pathways

CHAPTER 17 CONTROL OF BODY MOVEMENT

Module I: Local Control of Motor Neurons

Objectives

Upon completion of this module, the student will be able to:

1. Define *motor unit.*
2. Differentiate between spasticity, rigidity, and flaccidity.
3. Differentiate between voluntary and involuntary motor activities and state the role of learning in the development of involuntary responses.
4. Describe the monosynaptic stretch reflex by identifying each component in both anatomical terms and as elements of a negative-feedback control system for muscle length.
5. Describe the role of reciprocal innervation and activation of synergistic muscles in the knee jerk (see Fig. 17-3, p. 541).
6. Differentiate between alpha and gamma motor neurons.
7. Define and describe the significance of *alpha-gamma coactivation.*
8. Describe a Golgi tendon organ and state its function.

Reading Assignment

Chap. 17, pp. 537–544.

Exercises

Part I

Directions: Indicate a monosynaptic reflex in Fig. W-82 (p. 238). Use the symbols suggested. The only known monosynaptic reflex is the stretch reflex. Your answers should match A on Fig. 17-3, p. 541.

Part II

Directions: Indicate a polysynaptic reflex in Fig. W-83 (p. 239). Use the symbols suggested. As the text gives an example of the Golgi tendon organ, use *one* Golgi tendon organ, and the motor nerves to the two muscles. Check your answer against one of the Golgi tendon organ reflexes on Fig. 17-6, p. 544.

Part III

Directions: Complete Fig. W-84 (p. 240) to show the overall route of the Gamma loop. Circle the effects that occur in the muscle. (*543*)

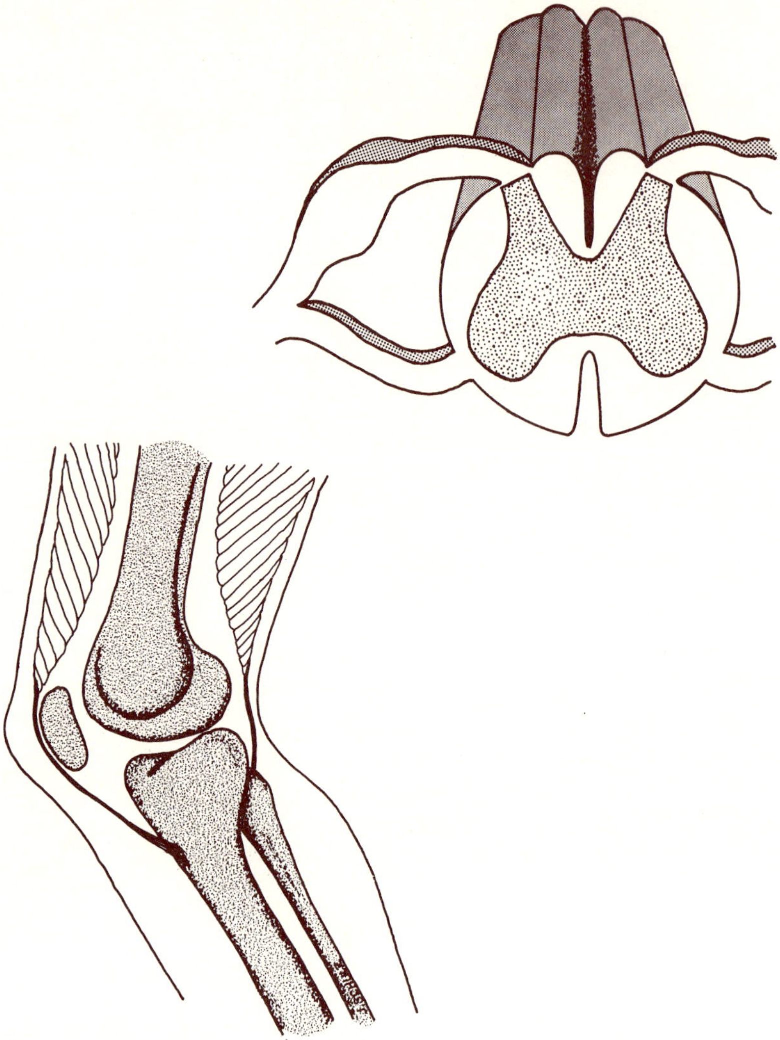

Fig. W-82 Monosynaptic reflex.

Key:

Muscle spindle

Afferent cell body

Motor nerve cell body

Excitatory synapse

Neuromuscular synapse

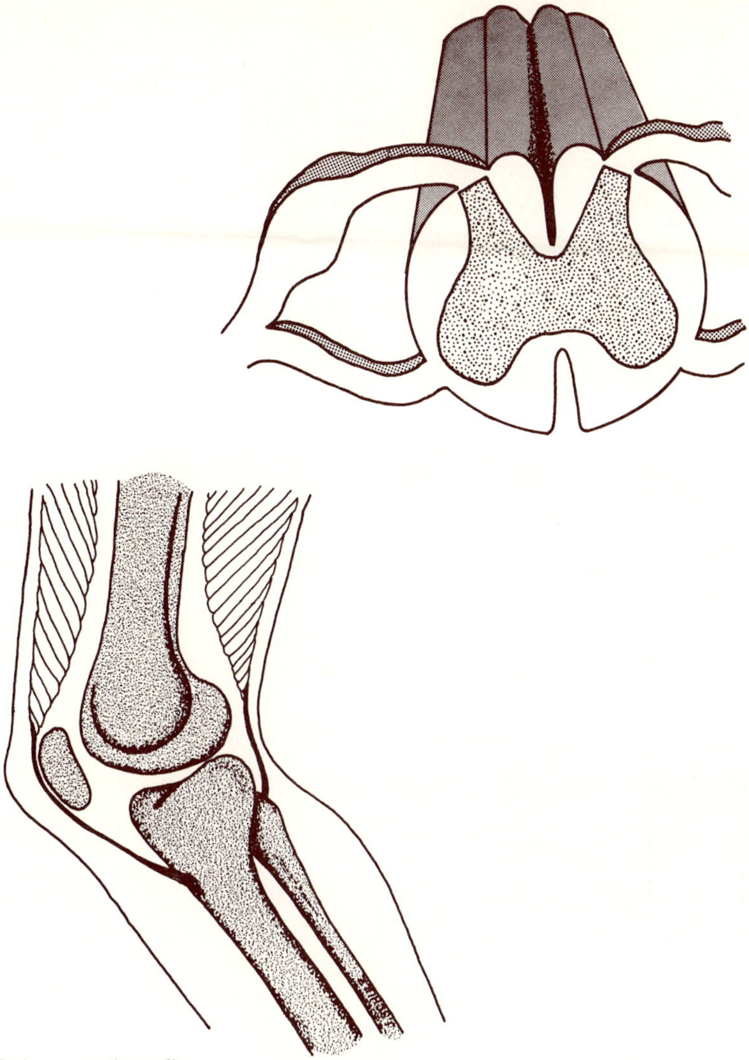

Fig. W-83 Polysynaptic reflex.

Key:

Golgi tendon organ

Afferent cell body

Interneuron cell body

Motor nerve cell body

Excitatory synapse

Inhibitory synapse

Neuromuscular synapse

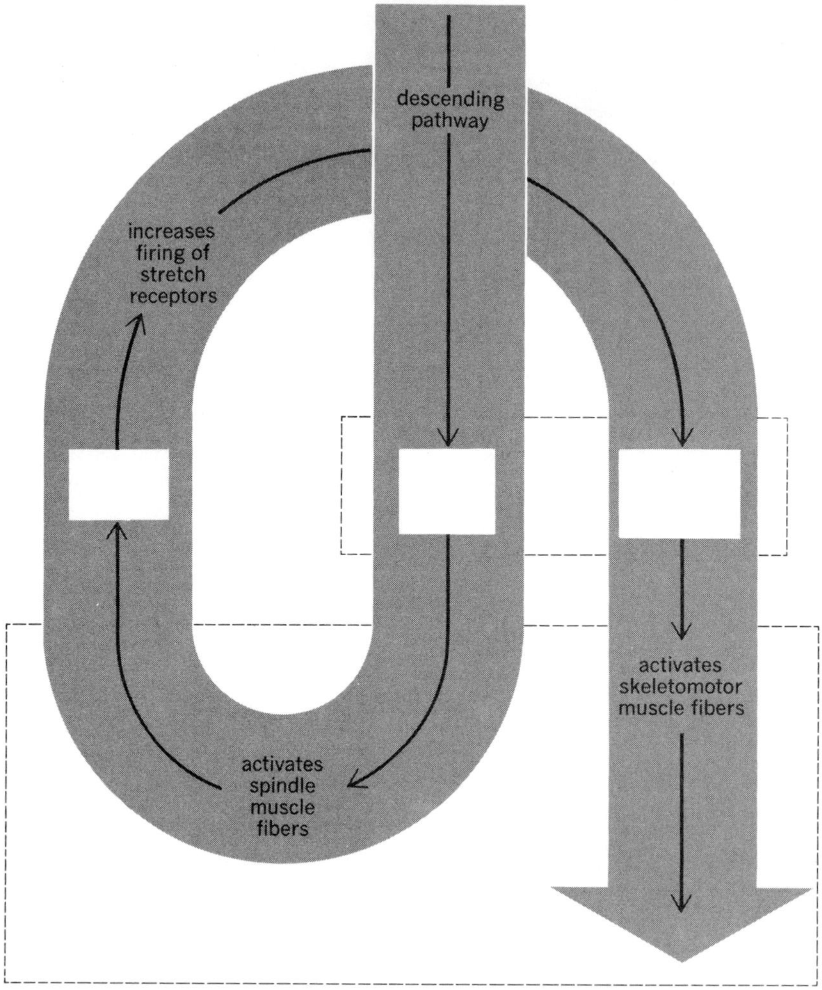

Fig. W-84 Descending pathway.

Self-Test

Part I

Directions: Circle the correct answer(s).

1. Flaccid muscles are

   a stiff. *b* weak. *c* awkward. *d* soft.

2. Which of the following structures are included in the gamma loop?

   a spindle muscle fiber
   b gamma motor neuron
   c alpha motor neuron
   d Golgi tendon organs

3. Almost all motor behavior
   a involves a conscious component.
   b involves an unconscious component.
   c is purely voluntary.
   d is purely involuntary.

Part II

Directions: Complete the following items in the space provided.

1. The excitation of one muscle and the simultaneous inhibition of its antagonistic muscle is called ________________.
2. The motor neurons controlling the skeletomotor muscle fibers are classified as ________________
3. Axons of what type of motor neurons innervate the spindle fibers? ________________

Part III

Directions: Circle T for true and F for false.

T F 1. The motor neurons which activate the spindle fibers are the same motor neurons which activate the skeletomotor muscle fibers.
T F 2. The gamma motor neurons are activated primarily by synaptic input from descending pathways.
T F 3. The selection of the specific pattern of neural activity is the function of centers in the spinal cord.
T F 4. The knee jerk is a good example of a negative-feedback control system.
T F 5. Stretch reflexes are the only known polysynaptic reflex arcs in man.

Module II: **Descending Pathways**

Objectives

Upon completion of this module, the student will be able to:

1. Describe three mechanisms by which descending pathways modify the activity of alpha motor neurons.
2. Differentiate between the direct corticospinal pathway and the multineuronal pathway in both anatomical and functional terms.
3. Describe the interactions of the motor cortex and subcortical centers in relation to coordination of muscle movement.

4. List the four general defects in movement that are associated with cerebellar damage.
5. Differentiate between the role of cortical input and general afferent input in the overall functioning of the cerebellum.
6. List one or more examples of the five components of the reflex arc (see p. 127) that would be involved in the maintenance of posture and balance.
7. List and describe the four components necessary for locomotion.

Reading Assignment

Chap. 17, pp. 544–552. Review Chap. 5, p. 127.

Exercises

Part I

Directions: Answer the following questions in the space provided.

1. You have a patient who got into an accident which resulted in some cerebellar damage. Keeping this in mind, answer the following questions.
   a How does the cerebellum affect the motor activity? ____________________

   ____

   b Does destruction of the cerebellum cause loss of any specific movement? __________

   c What kinds of problems might this patient suffer from? ____________________

   ______________________________________ *(547–548)*

Part II

Directions: Answer the following questions in the space provided.

The multineuronal pathway is a kind of descending pathway by which the cerebral cortex, subcortical centers, and cerebellum influence the motor neurons. Draw a simple diagram of the multineuronal pathway.

1. What kind of information does this pathway transmit? ____________________

   ____
2. Does the information that is transmitted by this pathway change or stay the same as it goes down through the cerebrum and brainstem? Why?
3. Is the multineuronal pathway functionally separated from the direct corticospinal pathway? Why? *(545–546)*

Part III

Directions: Complete the following chart by giving the name of the correct part of the brain according to the different properties. (*546–547*)

Properties	Name of the Correct Part of the Brain
Origin of descending pathways to motor neurons.	
Control of postural mechanisms, coordination of the simultaneous movements of locomotion.	
Voluntary control of slow, smooth movements.	
Influences the parts of the brain responsible for motor activity.	

Self-Test

Part I

Directions: Circle the correct answer(s).

1. The fibers of the direct corticospinal pathway end on

   a alpha motor neurons. *b* beta motor neurons.
   c gamma motor neurons. *d* interneurons.

2. The multineuronal motor pathway descending from the cortex synapses in the

   a basal ganglia.
   b brainstem nuclei.
   c brainstem reticular formation.
   d dorsal root ganglia.

3. The afferent inputs to the cerebellum come from which of the following?

   a eyes *b* skin *c* nose *d* joints

4. The postural reflexes occur whenever a person is

   a resting in bed. *b* walking on a rope.
   c rocking on a rocking chair. *d* falling.

Part II

Directions: Answer the following questions in the space provided.

1. What are the five components of the reflex arc?

   a ________________

   b ________________

   c ________________

   d ________________

   e ________________

2. Because of its shape in some parts of the brain, the direct corticospinal pathway is called

_________________________ or _________________________.

3. When a person with cerebellar damage tries to move his limbs, they go into oscillations.

This condition is known as _________________________ or

_________________________.

Part III

Directions: Circle T for true and F for false.

T F 1. The skeletal muscles on the left side of the body are controlled largely by neurons in the left half of the brain.

T F 2. The direct corticospinal pathway is the major mediator of fine movements.

T F 3. The basal ganglia serve a special role in the voluntary control of slow, smooth movements.

Module I:
Consciousness

Module II:
Behavior

CONSCIOUSNESS AND BEHAVIOR

CHAPTER 18

Module I: Consciousness

Objectives

Upon completion of this module, the student will be able to:

1. Match electroencephalogram (EEG) patterns with the five states of consciousness listed in Fig. 18-1, p. 554.
2. Define *epiphenomenon.*
3. Define *alpha rhythm* and state the subjective mood often associated with it.
4. Compare slow-wave sleep with paradoxical sleep in terms of EEG pattern, duration, ease of arousal, muscle tone, cardiovascular and respiratory state, and episodes of dreams.
5. Describe the reticular formation and reticular activating system.
6. Define *habituation.*
7. Describe the role of 5-HT (serotonin) in sleep.
8. Describe the role of sensory input in the maintenance of normal conscious experience.

Reading Assignment

Chapter 18, pp. 553–560.

Exercises

Part I

Directions: One way of defining various states of consciousness is by the characteristic EEG pattern. Sketch an EEG pattern for each of the states of consciousness shown in Fig. W-85. Artistic merit will not be judged, but pay particular attention to the features that differentiate the EEG patterns. (See Fig. 18-1, p. 554.)

Part II

Directions: States of consciousness are also identified by their behavioral aspects. Put an X in the appropriate spots of Chart I to indicate that a behavior is present in the state of consciousness listed. (See pp. 554–556.)

Chart I

Behavior	Alert	REM Sleep	Slow-Wave Sleep
Eyes open			
Eyes closed and relaxed			
Tonus in postural muscles			
Lack of tonus in postural muscles			
Irregular change in respiration, heart rate			
Easy to arouse			
Difficult to arouse			
Dreaming			

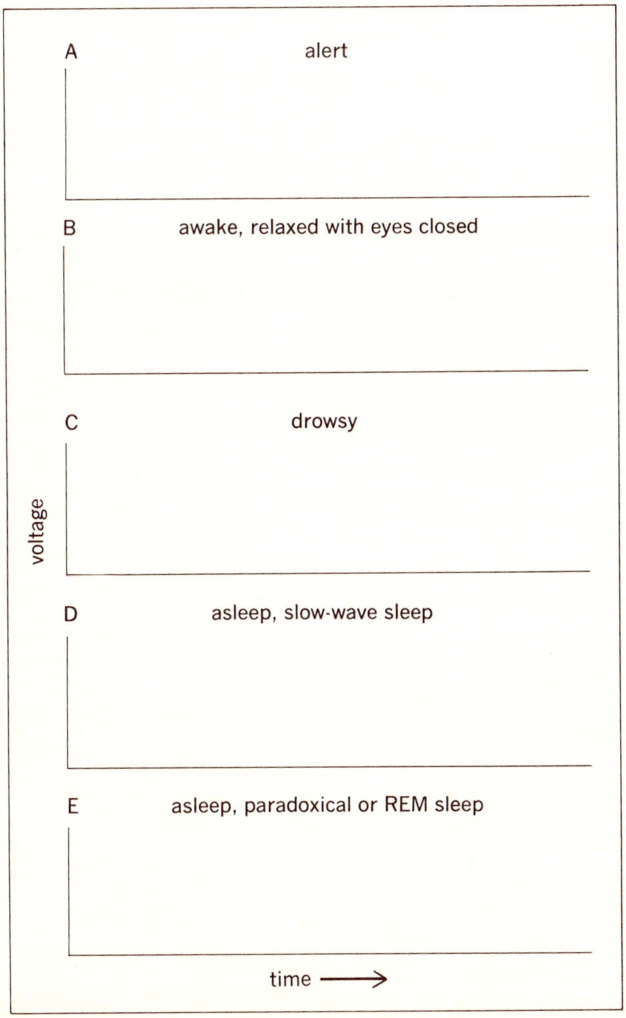

Fig. W-85

Part III

Directions: Define the following terms.

1. alpha rhythm (554)

2. epiphenomenon (554)

3. habituation (557)

Self-Test

Part I

Directions: Draw a series of graphs showing the voltages versus time for the five states of consciousness described in your text.

Part II

Directions: Circle the correct answer(s).

1. During the slow-wave sleep
   a the sleeper can be awakened easily.
   b dreams are more likely to occur than during paradoxical sleep.
   c muscle tone is inhibited.
   d respiration and heart rate are irregular.
2. Concerning the reticular activating system,
   a destruction of this area produces coma and the EEG pattern characteristic of the sleep state.
   b the neurons of the RAS activate the diffuse thalamic projection system.
   c the sensitivity of the RAS is selective, a phenomenon known as dishabituation.
   d amphetamines are thought to work by stimulating the RAS.
   e high levels of serotonin cause the excitation of the RAS, resulting in EEG patterns characteristic of paradoxical sleep.

Module II: Behavior

Objectives

Upon completion of this module, the student will be able to:

1. Define *motivation* in behavioral terms.
2. Describe reward and punishment in behavioral terms.
3. State the relation between goal-directed behavior, and reward and punishment directed behavior.
4. Describe a self-stimulation experiment.
5. State the relation between goal-directed behavior and the limbic system.
6. List the chemical transmitters known to be involved in subjective aspects of emotion/motivation as the biogenic amines norepinephrine and dopamine.
7. Describe the chemoaffinity theory of nerve connection development.
8. Describe the role of adequate nutrition and hormones in brain development.
9. State the role of the critical period in neural development.
10. Compare short-term with long-term memory.
11. Describe the molecular and morphological theories of memory.
12. Define *aphasia.*
13. State the role of the left cerebral hemisphere in language function.
14. Describe the language behavior of split-brain human beings.

Reading Assignment

Chap. 18, pp. 560–570.

Exercises

Part I

Directions: In self-stimulation experiments, electrical stimuli are delivered to specific parts of the brain through an implanted electrode. The results of such studies add to the knowledge of functions of particular areas of the brain. With this in mind, answer the following questions.

1. Is increased self-stimulation of a brain area punishing? ______________________

____

2. Are stimuli to some areas of the hypothalamus rewarding? ______________________

____

3. What indicates that this is so? ______________________
4. What areas of the hypothalamus are most closely related to highly rewarding self-stimulation? *(560–561)*

Part II

Directions: The two cerebral hemispheres are joined by commissures. When these nerve fiber bundles are severed, there are two separate mental domains: i.e., a "split brain." Keeping this in mind, answer each of the following questions.

1. Assuming the operation occurs after the age of twelve, which hemisphere is most likely to be found to control speech? ______________________ *(569)*
2. What does the development of essentially normal language in a split-brain child of five years old tell you about the critical period in neural development for speech? *(565)*

   ____

Part III

Directions: Answer the following questions in the space provided.

1. Describe the relationship between the hypothalamus and the limbic system. *(562–563)*

2. Adequate nutrition and hormones have an important role in brain development. Give an example to show the effect of decreased hormones during development. *(565)*

3. John wanted to get the phone number of the graduate school. He looked up the number in the directory, shut the directory and dialed the number.

   a What type of memory is this? ______________________

   b Which part of the brain is involved in this type of memory? ______________________

   c Is there an exclusive site for memory storage?

   ____

   d Does the removal of some parts of the brain remove specific memories? *(566)*

   ____

Self-Test

Part I

Directions: Complete the following statement.

1. The memory that exists during the time a memory trace is being laid down is called

   ______________________.

2. A language deficit in conceptualization or expression is called ____________________

____.

3. Retrograde amnesia, following unconsciousness, does not affect ____________________

____memory.

Part II

Directions: Circle the correct answer(s).

1. Which of the following structures are in part contained in the limbic system?

   a thalamus *b* hypothalamus
   c frontal cortex *d* pons
   e medulla

2. The limbic system is involved in

   a emotion. *b* fine motor movements.
   c vision. *d* arousal.

3. If the left hemisphere of the cerebral cortex is damaged, language may be permanently impaired if the damage occurs

   a before the age of two.
   b after age two and before age ten.
   c after age ten and before the early teens.
   d after the early teens.

4. Experiments which have located "rewarding" areas in the brain and which use implanted electrodes are called

   a split-brain experiments.
   b self-stimulation experiments.
   c neurosurgical experiments.
   d electrode experiments.

5. The "split-brain" studies have verified the fact that language functions occur in the

   a right cerebral hemisphere.
   b left cerebral hemisphere.

6. According to the chemoaffinity theory of neural development

   a certain neurons are attracted to each other.
   b during early development, neurons are capable of chemically identifying each other.
   c the precision of neural connections leads to highly specific synaptic connections.
   d the control of neural growth and development is entirely dependent on one's genetic code; environmental influences are unimportant.

Answer Key for Self-Tests

Chapter 1: Module I

Part I

1. liquid state *(13–14)*
2. water *(13–14)*
3. solute *(15)*
4. hydrogen *(14)*
5. hydrogen ions *(12)*

Part II

1. *c* *(15)*
2. *b* *(15)*

Part III

1. True *(7)*
2. True *(7)*
3. False. A proton has almost 2000 times the mass of an electron. *(7)*
4. False. Only as a liquid and gas. *(13–14)*
5. True *(15)*
6. False. Only for salts and substances with ionized or polar groups. *(15)*
7. False. Only those that ionize to form hydrogen ions. *(12)*
8. False. Neutral, polarized, or ionized molecules. *(13)*
9. True *(12–13)*
10. True *(7)*

Chapter 1: Module II

Part I

1. saturated *(25)*
2. triglyceride *(26)*
3. noncarbon molecules *(17)*
4. biochemistry *(17)*
5. polysaccharide *(28)*
6. disaccharide *(28)*
7. metabolism *(30)*
8. metabolic intermediates *(30)*
9. provides major source of energy *(29)*

Part II

1. *d* *(20)*
2. *c* *(20)*
3. *b* *(17–18)*
4. *b, c* *(19)*
5. *c* *(17)*
6. *c* *(28)*
7. *b* *(29)*
8. *b, e* *(26)*
9. *c* *(27)*
10. a *(26)*

Part III

1. E *(26)*
2. B *(21)*
3. D *(28)*
4. C *(27)*
5. A *(29)*

1. B *(20)*
2. D *(20)*
3. A *(20)*
4. C *(20)*

Chapter 2: Module I

Part I

1. *a, c* *(39)*
2. *a* *(35)*
3. *a, c* *(35)*

Part II

1. True. Molecules move back and forth with net movement in only one direction. *(38)*
2. True *(38)*
3. False. Diffusion. *(38)*
4. False. Diffusion. *(39)*
5. False. There is movement of particles in both directions but there is no net flux. *(39)*

Part III

1. higher, lower *(38)*
2. flux *(38)*
3. concentration *(38)*
4. $F_B = K_B \Delta P$ *(35)*
5. $F = K_P(C_o - C_i)$ *(41)*
6. large *(42)*
7. $F = K(C_1 - C_2)$ *(39)*

Chapter 2: Module II

Part I

1. True *(43)*
2. False. For large or polar molecules. *(43)*
3. False. Carrier molecule is confined to the membrane. *(43)*
4. False. From high to low concentration. *(46)*

Part II

1. osmolarity *(50)*
2. phagocytosis *(49)*
3. fluid, solid *(49)*
4. osmosis *(49)*
5. penetrating *(53)*

6. saturated (43)
7. specificity (43)
8. hypertonic (53)
9. decreases (53)
10. *a* 1
    b 2
    c 3 (53)

Part III

1. *a* D (38)
   b B (35)
   c D (38)
   d M (47)
   e D (49)
   f M (43)
2. *a* H
   b I
   c H
   d O
   e O (53)
3. *d* (47)
4. *c* (43)
5. a, c (44)

Chapter 2: Module III

Part I

1. False. The major lipids are phospholipids. (54)
2. True (56)
3. False. Fatty-acid chains interact with one another. (55)
4. False. At a gap junction, this occurs. (59)
5. True (60)
6. True (54)

Part II

1. *c* (56)
2. *a, c* (54)

Part III

1. fatty acids (54)
2. protein, lipid, protein (55)
3. a desmosome (58)
4. tight junction (59)
5. *a* D (58)
   b G (59)
   c T (59)
   d G (60)
   e D (58)

Chapter 3: Module I

Part I

Skim chapter for italicized words if you missed any in Part I.

1. *c*
2. *f*
3. *d*
4. *e*
5. *h*
6. *i*
7. *g*
8. *a*
9. *b*

Part II

1. Raising the concentration of any one molecule species in a chemical reaction increases the rate at which that molecule undergoes a reaction with other molecules in the system and thus alters the concentration of both product and reactant molecules. (64)
2. Activation energy is the energy that must be supplied to a molecule to break the chemical or electrical forces holding that molecule together. (65; see especially Fig. 3-2)
3. One way to alter the activity of an enzyme is by changing the shape of its active site. A modulator molecule combines with the enzyme (allosteric enzyme) at a site distant from the active site; however, in the process, the active site is altered, changing the enzyme's activity. A second way enzyme activity is altered is by the presence or absence of coenzymes, the low-molecular weight substances required for activity of many enzymes. (70)
4. Substrate + enzyme → enzyme − substrate complex → product + enzyme (66)

Part III

1. *a, b, c, d, e* (63–66)
2. *a, d* (66)
3. *a, b, d* (65)
4. *b, c* (70)

Chapter 3: Module II

Part I

1. mitochondria, oxidative phosphorylation (74)
2. The energy yield of triglyceride is 0.55 mole of ATP/g (463 ATP/842 g). The energy yield of glucose is 0.21 mole of ATP/g (38 ATP/180 g). (86)
3. hydrogen, water, ATP (74–76)
4. Krebs cycle, mitochondria (81)

Part II

1. *a, b, c, d, e* (74–77)
2. *a, c* (78–80)
3. *a, b, d* (87–89)

Part III

1. True (80)
2. False (83)
3. True (83)
4. True (86)
5. True (89)

Chapter 4: Module I

Part I

Skim chapter for italicized words if you missed any in Part I.

1. a
2. *a, d, f*
3. *c*
4. *d*
5. *d, h*
6. *c*
7. *f*
8. *f*
9. *h*

Part II

1. *d* (*97–102*)
2. *c* (*97*)
3. *a, b, c, f* (*94–95*)
4. *a, b, c, e, g, i* (*95–97*)
5. *a, b, c* (remember, uracil replaces thymine in RNA) (*97–99*)
6. *e* (*103*)
7. *a, b, c* (*108–109*)
8. *a, b, c, d, e, f* (*109*)

Part III

1. lysosome (*106*)
2. polyribosome (*103*)
3. secretory granules (*104*)
4. *a* on DNA surface by regulating the ability to synthesize a specific mRNA
   b at the ribosome level by modifying the ability of mRNA to combine with the ribosome, the movement of the ribosome along mRNA, or the activity of the various ribosomal enzymes
   c by controlling the dynamic equilibrium of mRNA (i.e., rate of synthesis/breakdown)
   d regulating synthesis of tRNA and rRNA on DNA (*107–108*)

Chapter 4: Module II

Part I

1. *c* (*111*)
2. *a, d, e* (*111–113*)
3. *a, b, c* (*113–114*)
4. *a, b, c, e, f, g* (*115*)
5. *b, d, f* (*117*)
6. *c, d, f* (*117*)

Chapter 5: Module I

Part I

1. False. It is highly sensitive to extracellular fluid. (*122*)
2. True (*123*)
3. False. There are marked differences in concentration. (*123*)

Part II

1. homeostasis (*123*)
2. chemical evolution (*121*)
3. sodium (*122*)
4. proteinoids (*121*)
5. interstitial fluid plasma (*123*)

Part III

A, B, B, A, (*123*)

Chapter 5: Module II

Part I

1. False. Can maintain steady state by restoring a variable toward a set point. (*126*)
2. True (*128*)
3. False. As receptor and integrating center. Bone is the effector. (*128*)

Part II

1. *b* (*129*)
2. *c* (*126*)
3. *b* (*127*)
4. *a, d* (*127*)

Chapter 5: Module III

Part I

1. *a* (*132*)
2. *b, c* (*131*)
3. *c* (*131*)

Part II

1. positive balance (*131*)
2. menstrual cycle (*132*)
3. net loss/net gain (in either order) (*130*)

Part III

1. False. Relatively constant. (*132*)
2. False. Varies with many factors. (*132*)
3. True (*131*)

Chapter 6: Module I

Part I

1. False. It varies from 5 to 100 mV. (*136*)
2. True (*136*)
3. False. The chloride ion is not actively transported as are sodium and potassium. (*139*)
4. False. The water compartments of the body contain many charged particles and therefore are good conductors. (*136*)
5. True (*136*)
6. False. It is 50 to 75 times more permeable to potassium. (*138*)

Part II

1. *c* (*136*)
2. *c* (*139*)
3. *b* (*135*)
4. *a, d* (*135*)

Chapter 6: Module II

Part I

1. True (*142*)
2. False. It is becoming depolarized. (*140*)
3. False. It results from a change in membrane permeabilities. Concentration gradients do not change. (*141*)
4. True (*141*)
5. False. Threshold potential is closer to zero than resting membrane potential. (*140*)

Part II

1. excitability (*140*)
2. subthreshold stimulus (*142*)
3. 600 (*141*)
4. sodium inactivation (*141*)
5. all or none (*143*)

Chapter 6: Module III

Part I

1. False. It can be stimulated but will produce no action potential. (*144*)
2. False. The action potential leaps from one node to the next in the myelinated fibers. (*146*)
3. True (*146*)
4. True (*144*)
5. False. They are transmitted without decrement. (*145*)

Part II

1. *a, c* (*146*)
2. *b, e* (*144*)
3. *a, b* (*146*)

Chapter 6: Module IV

Part I

1. unchanged (*149–150*)
2. receptor (*149–150*)
3. frequency (*151*)
4. adaptation (*152*)
5. recruitment (*153*)

Part II

1. False. They are graded. (*152*)
2. True (*149*)
3. False. They are a graded response and may increase in size. (*151*)
4. False. A generator potential has no refractory period. (*152*)
5. True (*147*)

Part II

1. *c, d* (*152*)
2. *a, b* (*152*)
3. *a, d* (*149–150*)

Chapter 6: Module V

Part I

1. *b, c* (*160*)
2. *b* (*157*)
3. *c* (*156*)

Part II

1. True (*157*)
2. False. Serotonin is a synaptic transmitter. (*159*)
3. False. An IPSP causes a hyperpolarization. (*156*)
4. False. They last more than 10 times as long. (*158*)
5. True (*161*)

Part III

1. synaptic vesicle (*155*)
2. spatial summation (*158*)
3. neuroeffector transmitters (*160*)
4. transmitter receptor sites (*160*)
5. presynaptic inhibition (*160*)

Chapter 6: Module VI

Part I

1. True (*164*)
2. False. Somatic efferent neurons go directly to the effector organs without synapse. (*165*)
3. False. At the effector organ, sympathetic fibers release norepinephrine. (*164*)
4. True (*166*)
5. False. It decreases both rate and contractility. (*suppl.*)

Part II

1. craniosacral (*164*)
2. white matter (*166*)
3. parasympatholytic (*164*)
4. reciprocal innervation (*164*)
5. brainstem (*167*)

Part III

1. *b* (*suppl.*)
2. *a, d* (*suppl.*)
3. *c* (*169*)
4. *b* (*168*)

Chapter 7: Module I

Part I

1. False. Hormones secreted by endocrine glands act by these mechanisms; secretions from exocrine glands do not. *(172–176)*
2. True *(177)*
3. False *(177)*
4. True *(177)*
5. True *(177)*
6. False. Some endocrine diseases lead to pharmacological effects from the "oversecreted" hormone. *(178)*

Part II

1. all correct *(177–178)*
2. *a, c, e, f* *(178)*

Chapter 7: Module II

Part I

1. *b, d* *(179)*
2. *a, b* *(179)*
3. *c, d* *(180)*
4. *c, d* *(184)*

Part II

1. *a* posterior lobe *(180)*
   b anterior lobe *(180)*
2. hypothalamopituitary portal system *(183)*
3. Neurons located in the hypothalamus are believed to terminate around the hypothalamic capillary origins of portal vessels connecting the hypothalamus to the anterior pituitary. The neurons secrete substances into the capillaries. These substances are carried by the portal vessels to the anterior pituitary where they stimulate release of certain hormones. *(183)*
4. A releasing factor influences the release of a specific hormone from the anterior pituitary. *(183)*
5. *a* TSH-releasing factor
   b ACTH-releasing factor
   c FSH-releasing factor
   d LH-releasing factor
   e GH-releasing factor
   f Prolactin-inhibiting factor *(184)*
6. See Fig. W-13, p. 257. *(184)*

Part III

See Table A-1, p. 257.

Part IV

1. False. The posterior pituitary is an outgrowth of the hypothalamus *(185)*
2. False. The neurons are located within the hypothalamic nuclei some distance from the posterior pituitary. *(185)*
3. True *(185)*
4. True *(185)*

Chapter 8: Module I

Part I

1. True. Connective tissue surrounding individual cells carries the blood vessels and nerve fibers. *(190)*
2. False. Collagen has no contractile properties. *(190)*
3. True. The different bands cause the light and dark striated appearance. *(190)*

Part II

1. smooth *(189–190)*
2. six *(192)*
3. myosin, actin *(193)*

Part III

1. *a, b, c* *(195)*
2. *b* *(195)*

Part IV

1. bridge contraction *(194)*
2. actin binding *(194)*
3. bridge relaxation *(194)*

Chapter 8: Module II

Part I

1. True *(198)*
2. True *(209)*
3. True *(198)*
4. False. There is maximal overlap for developing tension. *(209)*
5. True *(201)*
6. False. The esterase is part of the motor end plate. *(202)*
7. False. Very nearly l_0, and this is the optimal length. *(209)*

Part II

1. sarcolemma or muscle membrane *(196)*
2. neuromuscular or myoneural *(199)*
3. acetylcholine *(202)*
4. brain and spinal cord *(202)*
5. summation *(206)*
6. motor unit *(201)*

Part III

1. *b* *(197)*
2. *b* *(195)*

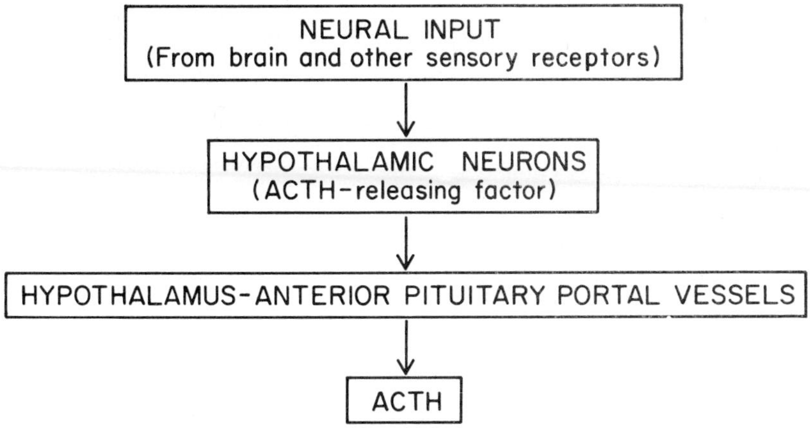

(184)

Fig. W-13

Table A-1

Events	Effects on Rates of Secretion of: Releasing Hormones	Pituitary Hormones	Target Gland Hormones
1. Hypothalamic lesions	Falls to 0	All decrease (except for prolactin)	Decreases
2. Pituitary destruction	Increases	Decreases	Decreases
3. Pituitary transplantation to a distant site in the body	Increases	Decreases (except for prolactin)	Decreases
4. Increase in pituitary hormone secretion	Decreases		Increases
5. Decrease in pituitary hormone secretion	Increases		Decreases

(184–185)

3. *b* *(195)*
4. *c* *(204)*
5. *c* *(208)*

Part IV

1. Isometrics; "tension" should be circled. *(205)*
2. Isotonic; "distance shortened" should be circled. *(205)*

Chapter 8: Module III

Part I

1. hypertrophy *(216)*
2. *a* by transformation of one biochemical type of fiber into another
   b by the growth in size of the muscle fibers *(219)*
3. denervation atrophy *(216)*
4. disuse atrophy *(216)*
5. pacemaker potential *(223)*
6. *a* creatine phosphate
   b substrate phosphorylation during glycolysis
   c oxidative phosphorylation in the mitochondria *(213)*

Part II

1. True *(221)*
2. True *(225)*

3. False. Myosin ATPase breaks down ATP at a very rapid rate. *(214)*
4. True *(214)*

Part III

1. *a, b, d* *(225)*
2. *a* *(214)*
3. *b, c, d* *(218)*
4. *a, b, c* *(216)*

Chapter 9: Module I

Part I

1. *a* oxygen
   b carbon dioxide
   c nutrients
   d wastes
   (Other substances are also carried, as indicated by Objective 1.) *(229)*
2. Fig. 9-1, p. 230, and Fig. W-20, p. 259
3. four (aortic, pulmonary, and two atrioventricular valves) *(231)*
4. See Fig. 9-3, p. 232.

Part II

1. False. The hematocrit is the percentage of total blood volume which is *cells.* *(228)*
2. False. The total blood volume of a 70-kg person is between 5 and 6 liters. *(229)*

Chapter 9: Module II

Part I

1. See Fig. 9-10, p. 236.
2. See Fig. W-25, p. 259 *(238)*

Part II

1. False. Blood does not flow during isovolumetric ventricular contraction. *(239–240)*
2. True. There is continuous flow. *(240)*
3. False. Ventricles can contract without being excited from the SA node during conditions such as asynchrony or fibrillation. *(235)*

Part III

See Fig. W-26, p. 260. *(239)*

Chapter 9: Module III

Part I

See Chart A-1, p. 260. *(241–242)*

Part II

1. False. A decrease in flow would tend to produce a decrease in intraventricular pressure and a decrease in ventricular distension, and thus a corresponding decrease in stroke volume. *(242)*
2. False. This statement would be true for the stimulation of the sympathetic nerves, not the parasympathetic nerves. *(241)*
3. True. SV is determined by end diastolic volume which in turn can be increased by either increasing intraventricular pressure or decreasing intrathoracic pressure, or both. *(244)*
4. False. Even though the patient's stroke volume falls in a normal range, the ventricles may be over- or underdistended through the beat. To answer this question you must know the actual end-diastolic or end-systolic volumes. *(244)*

Chapter 9: Module IV

Part I

1. R_1 = 0.5 mmHg/ml/min

$$F = \frac{\Delta P}{R}$$

$$R = \frac{\Delta P}{F} = \frac{81 - 76}{10} = \frac{5}{10} = 0.5$$

If R_1 = 0.5 mmHg/ml/min and R_2 is for a vessel two times as long, then R_2 = 1 mmHg/ml/min

$$F = \frac{\Delta P}{R} = \frac{5}{1} = 5 \text{ ml/min}$$

a 1 ml/min · mmHg
b 1 mmHg/ml · min
c 5 ml/min *(246–247)*

Part II

1. True. The artery diameters are so large they have essentially no effect on pressure. *(249)*
2. False. They have no muscle in their walls. *(255)*
3. False. The arterioles control capillary blood flow. *(251)*
4. False. The resistance is lower which helps reduce the pressure. The pressure entering the lungs from the heart is lower than the pressure entering the systemic circulation. *(239)*

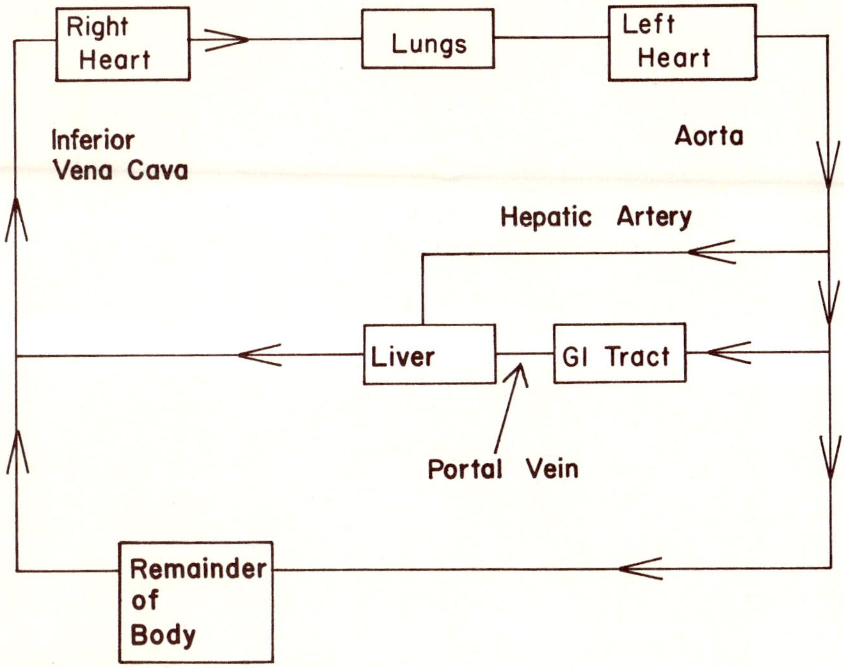

Fig. W-20

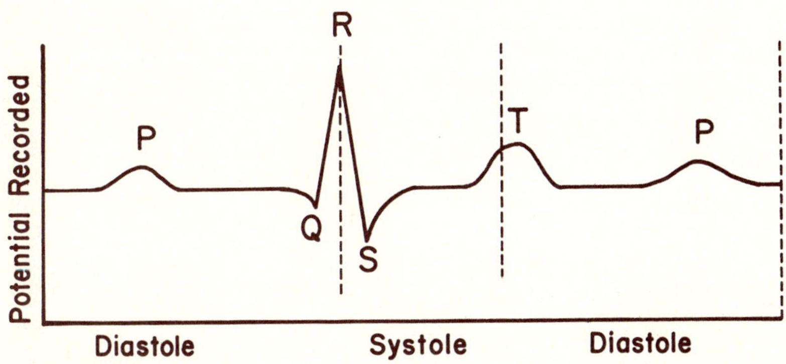

Fig. W-25

Chapter 9: Module V

Part I

1. False. Resistance changes in arterioles cause a rise or fall in capillary hydrostatic blood pressure. *(258–259)*
2. False. Difference in water concentration causes fluid to flow into the capillaries at the venule end. *(258)*
3. False. Capillaries are relatively impermeable to proteins. *(257)*
4. True *(260)*

Part II

All blanks should be checked. *(252–254)*

Part III

1. *a, b* *(263)*
2. *b* *(253)*

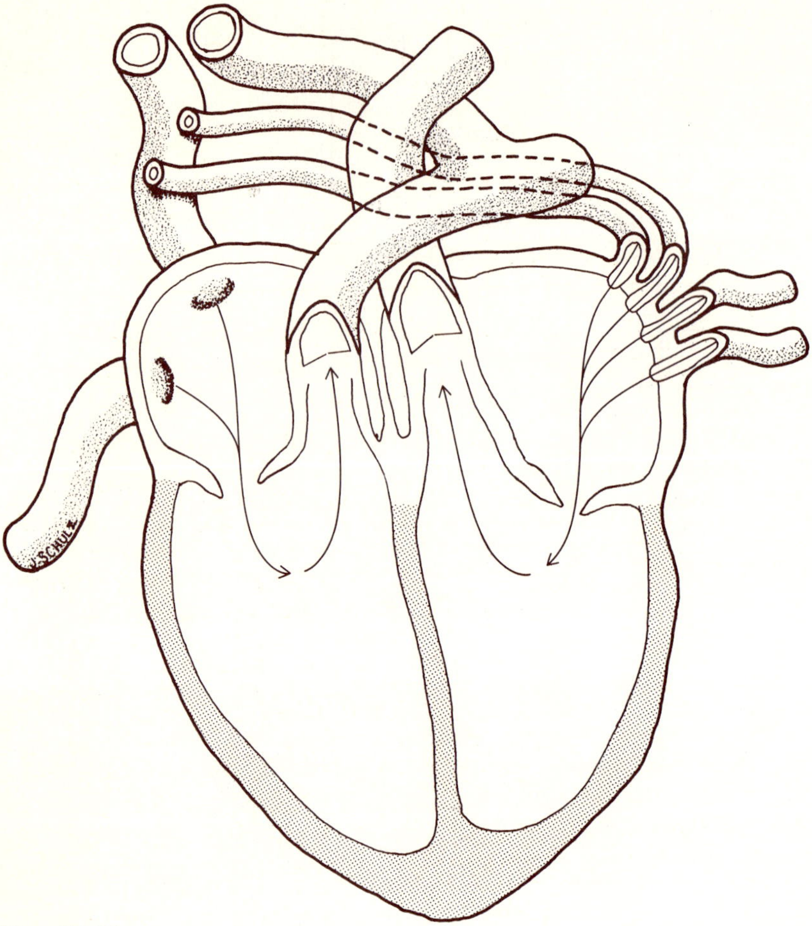

Fig. W-26

Chart A-1

	HR	× *SV*	= *CO*
1.	↔	↑	↑
2.	↓	↔	↓
3.	↑	↑	↑
4.	↔	↓	↓
5.	↑	↑	↑

3. *c* (*253*)
4. *a* (*257*)
5. *a* (*263*)

Part IV

1. increase
2. increase
3. decrease
4. decrease (*258–259*)

Chapter 9: Module VI

Part I

1. False. Some will, but not usually all. In particular, the heart and brain rarely have reduced blood flows. (*265*)
2. False. Hyperemia is increased blood flow in response to increased activity of tissues. (*252*)
3. True. Increasing arteriole diameter decreases total peripheral resistance and

leads to a decrease in blood pressure. (267)
4. False. They start firing slower. (269)
5. True. The body generally cannot significantly change the length of the vessels. (247)
6. True. The pulmonary arterioles are excluded in determining TPR. (267)

Part II

3–top, 1–middle, 2–bottom (269–270)

Part III

1. ↑, ↓
2. ↓, ↑
3. ↑, ↓
4. ↑, ↓ (271)

Part IV

See Chart A-2, p. 262 of workbook, and see p. 271, Fig. 9-51.

Chapter 9: Module VII

Part I

1. *c* (271)
2. *b* (273)
3. *a, c* (275)
4. *a, c* (277)
5. *c* (273)

Part II

1. *a, c* (281)

Chapter 10: Module I

Part I

1. respiratory system (284)
2. ventilation (287)
3. respiration (284)

Part II

See Figs. 10-1 and 10-2, pp. 284–285.

Part III

1. False. The cilia line the respiratory tract. (285)
2. False. The cilia start at the trachea. (285)
3. True. The mucus and entrapped particles are deposited in the pharynx to be swallowed or expectorated. (285)
4. False. The fluid fills the pleural cavity outside the alveoli. (287)
5. True. The paralysis of the cilia by agents such as cigarette smoke may lead to lung infections. (285)

Part IV

1. The only correct answer is *c*. Answer *a*, bulk flow, describes the movement of air from the atmosphere to the lungs. (287)

Chapter 10: Module II

Part I

1. pneumothorax (288)
2. intrapleural (287)
3. bulk flow or ventilation (287)
4. vital capacity (293)
5. residual volume (293)
6. tidal volume (293)
7. expiratory reserve volume (293)
8. inspiratory reserve volume (293)
9. vital capacity (293)
10. pulmonary surfactant (295)
11. minute ventilatory volume (293)
12. anatomic (293)
13. dead space (294)
14. 1100 ml (293)

Part II

1. *c*, synonymous with (289)
2. *a* (289)
3. active, passive (289)
4. *b, c* (290)

Part III

1. CO_2, O_2 (292)
2. residual volume, 1000 ml (293)
3. reserve volume, 2500–3500 ml, 1000 ml (293)
4. tidal volume, 500 ml (293)
5. resting tidal volume, inspiratory reserve, expiratory reserve (293)
6. Chart I

   a 6000

   b 6000

   c 6000

   d 6000

   Chart II

   a 6000:(150) × (40)
   b 2400
   c 6000: (150) × (12)
   d 6000 (294)

Part IV

1. False. The volume of the conducting airways which cannot exchange gas is known as the anatomic dead space (293)
2. True (295)
3. False. Pneumothorax is the condition that exists when the chest wall is pierced and atmospheric air rushes into the intrapleural space.

Chart A-2

	↑ Parasympathetic	↑ Sympathetic
HR	↓	↑
Total peripheral resistance	↔	↑
CO	↓	↑
Blood flow to viscera	↔	↓

Under these conditions, the lungs collapse. *(288)*

4. False. Asthma is characterized by severe bronchiolar smooth muscle constriction and plugging of the airways by bronchial secretions. This condition causes a decrease in anatomic dead space. *(291)*

Chapter 10: Module III

Part I

1. $RQ = \frac{CO_2 \text{ produced}}{O_2 \text{ consumed}}$ *(296)*
2. 1.0, 0.7 *(296)*
3. concentration + speed of molecules *(297)*
4. diffusion *(297)*
5. *a* PO_2 in gas
   b solubility of O_2 in liquid *(297)*
6. Your answer should indicate that this is due to the large amount of air left in the lungs after expiration. "Just because" is *not* an adequate answer. *(298)*
7. *a* physically dissolved in the blood, 1 to 3 percent
   b chemically bound to hemoglobin, 97 to 99 percent (Note that the sum of your percents should be 100 percent) *(299)*
8. *a* physically dissolved in blood, 8 percent
   b chemically bound to hemoglobin, 25 percent
   c converted into bicarbonate and hydrogen ions, 67 percent *(305)*
9. carbonic anhydrase *(305)*
10. hydrogen ions and bicarbonate ions *(305)*
11. Any two of the following are correct: a functional reduction in the number of alveoli, as in emphysema; a thickening of alveolar walls; a functional thickening of alveolar walls, as in edema; a formation of denser, less permeable alveolar walls, as caused by inhalation of beryllium *(298, 316)*

Part II

1. >
2. >
3. <
4. <
5. <
6. > *(298)*

Part III

1. M *(303)*
2. H *(299)*
3. M and H *(303)*
4. neither *(303)*

Chapter 10: Module IV

Part I

1. *c* *(307)*
2. *a, c, e* *(307–308)*
3. *b, d* *(310)*
4. *b* *(310)*
5. *d* *(312)*
6. *e* *(313–314)*

Part II

1. *a* carotid body
   b aortic body *(310)*
2. increases, decreased *(312)*
3. hyperventilation *(311)*
4. hypoventilation *(311)*
5. apnea *(311)*

Part III

1. False. Blood cells are produced only in the marrow. *(317)*
2. True. (4 months) × (30 days/month) = 120 days. *(316)*
3. False. Sorry. The process is erythropoiesis; the hormone that stimulates it is erythropoietin. *(317–318)*
4. True *(317)*
5. False. Hemoglobin is broken down to bilirubin; O_2 combines with the iron. *(317)*
6. False. This is a half-truth. Iron balance is maintained by the intestinal epithelium. *(317–318)*
7. True *(316)*

8. True (318)
9. False. The erythrocyte is broken down by phagocytes. (317)
10. True (316)

Chapter 11: Module I

Part I

1. Regulation of extracellular water and electrolytes (320)
2. *a* H_2O
   b Na^+
   c Ca^{2+}
   d K^+
   e H^+ (in any order) (320)
3. Check Fig. 11-1, p. 321, for correct labeling.

Part II

Check Figs. 11-2 and 11-3, p. 322, for correct labeling.

Chapter 11: Module II

Part I

1. *a, c, d* (328)
2. *c* (325)
3. *d* (325)
4. *a* (325)

Part II

Substance B—filtered, secreted, not reabsorbed; Substance C—filtered, partially reabsorbed; Substance D—filtered, totally reabsorbed (324)

Part III

1. Characteristics: filtered at the glomerulus but not secreted or reabsorbed; all of filtered amount appears in the urine.
   Example: inulin (326)
2. GFR = 200 liters/day

   GFR liters/day

   $$= \frac{\text{mg/liter} \times \text{liters/day}}{\text{mg/liter}}$$

   $$= \frac{350 \text{ mg/liter} \times 2 \text{ liters/day}}{3.5 \text{ mg/liter}}$$

   (326)
3. RPF = 1,000 liters/day

   RPF = 200 liters/day × 5 (326)
4. 9 g

   Excreted = filtered − reabsorbed
   = 0.05 g/liter × 180 liters/day − 0
   = 9 g/day (326)
5. *c.* clearance units are volume/time, not mass/time (326)
6. *a.* $C_{In} = \frac{U_{In} \times V}{P_{In}}$

   $= 100$ mg/100 ml

   $$= \frac{\times 1.4 \text{ liters/day}}{1 \text{ mg/100 ml}}$$

   = 140 liters/day

   $$C_{urea} = \frac{U_{urea} \times V}{P_{urea}}$$

   = 220 m*M*/liter

   $$= \frac{\times 1.4 \text{ liters/day}}{5 \text{ m}M\text{/liter}}$$

   = 61.6 liters/day

   $$C_{PAH} = \frac{U_{PAH} \times V}{PAH}$$

   $$= \frac{700 \text{ mg/ml} \times 1.4 \text{ liters/day}}{2 \text{ mg/ml}}$$

   = 490 liters/day

   b. Reabsorbed urea:
   = filtered urea − excreted urea
   = 140 liters/day × 5 m*M*/liter − 220 mg/ml × 1.4 liters/day
   = 392 m*M*/day

   c. PAH secreted:
   = PAH excreted − PAH filtered
   = 700 mg/ml × 1.4 liters/day − 2 mg/ml × 140 liters/day
   = 980 g/day − 280 g/day
   = 700 g/day (325–326)
7. No change.

   $$C_{In} = \frac{U_{In} \times V}{P_{In}}$$

   When P_{In} increases, there is no change in C_{In} because U_{In} rises an identical amount, i.e., the mass of inulin filtered and excreted increases but the volume of plasma supplying this inulin is increased. In the process, the plasma becomes cleared of inulin. (326)
8. *a* Substance A is a large molecule poorly filtered at the glomerulus.
   b Substance A is bound, at least in part, to plasma protein.
   c Substance A is reabsorbed. (326)
9. *a* This waste product is normally excreted in large amounts. A decreased GFR would cause its plasma concentrations to increase until a filtered load was increased enough to reestablish normal excretion. In contrast, the reabsorption T_m's for glucose, amino acids, purines, and other organic compounds which are not waste products, are usually so high as to prevent significant excretion. Their plasma concentrations are virtually independent of the renal function; for ex-

ample, the kidneys do not participate in the "setting" of their plasma concentrations. (327–328)

Chapter 11: Module III

Part I

See Chart A-3.

Part II

1. *a, b, c* (Water and chloride are reabsorbed passively as a result of electrochemical gradients generated by active sodium reabsorption. Urea is reabsorbed passively as a result of concentration gradients established by water reabsorption and indirectly by sodium reabsorption. Glucose has its own active transport system.) (332)
2. *a, b, c, d* (340–343)
3. *c, d, e* (334)
4. *a, b* (*c* is untrue because the impulses from increased atrial pressure *inhibit* not stimulate the ADH-producing cells. *d* is untrue because it is the converse of *c*). (337)
5. *a, b, d, e* (343)
6. *b, c, d, g, h, i, j, l* (339–340)

Chapter 11: Module IV

Part I

1. *b, e* (353)
2. *a, b, d* (354)

Part II

1. calcium concentration of the plasma (347–349)
2. phosphoric and sulfuric acids, organic acids, carbonic acid (H_2CO_3) and H^+ dissociation to bicarbonate (HCO_3^-) (350–351)

Part III

1. True (346)
2. False. It has just the opposite effect. (347)
3. False. By parathormone and by calcitonin. (349)
4. False. It is controlled directly by the calcium concentration of the extracellular fluid bathing the cells of the parathyroid glands. There are *no* intermediary hormones or nerves. (347)
5. False. Are opposing, but control calcium levels. (347–349)
6. True (348)
7. False. Only the kidneys actually eliminate hydrogen ions. The lungs allow the escape of CO_2 which reverses the process of association with water to form carbonic acid. (351)
8. True (351)
9. True (353)
10. False. Mostly by tubular secretion only. (353)
11. True (352–353)

Part IV

1. *a, f*
2. *c*
3. *b, e, f*
4. *d*
5. *e*
6. *d*
7. *e, f*
8. *e, f*
9. *g*
10. *f* (349–353)

Part V

1. *a, d, e, f, h* (345–346)
2. *b, e* (347–348)
3. *c, d, e* (350–351)
4. *a, b, c* (351–352)

Chapter 12: Module I

Part I

See Fig. 12-1, p. 356.

Part II

See Fig. W-54.

Part III

1. *a* external autonomic nerves
   b internal plexus nerve fibers
   c hormones secreted by GI tract itself (358)
2. *a* parotid
   b submaxillary (submandibular)
   c sublingual (359)
3. *a* food products
   b acid
   c volume
   d osmolarity (360)

Part IV

1. *a, b, d* (359–361)
2. *b, c* (361)
3. *c, d, e* (362)
4. *b* (363)

Part V

1. False. In actuality, humans need to chew food only if the particles are too large to be swallowed. (359)
2. True. The smell and sight of food are just two examples. (360)

Chart A-3

GFR	Na Reabsorption	Na Excretion	Cl Excretion	H_2O Excretion
N	D	I	I	I
N	I	D	D	D
I	D	I	I	I
I	I	D, N, or I	D, N, or I	D, N, or I

(331–333)

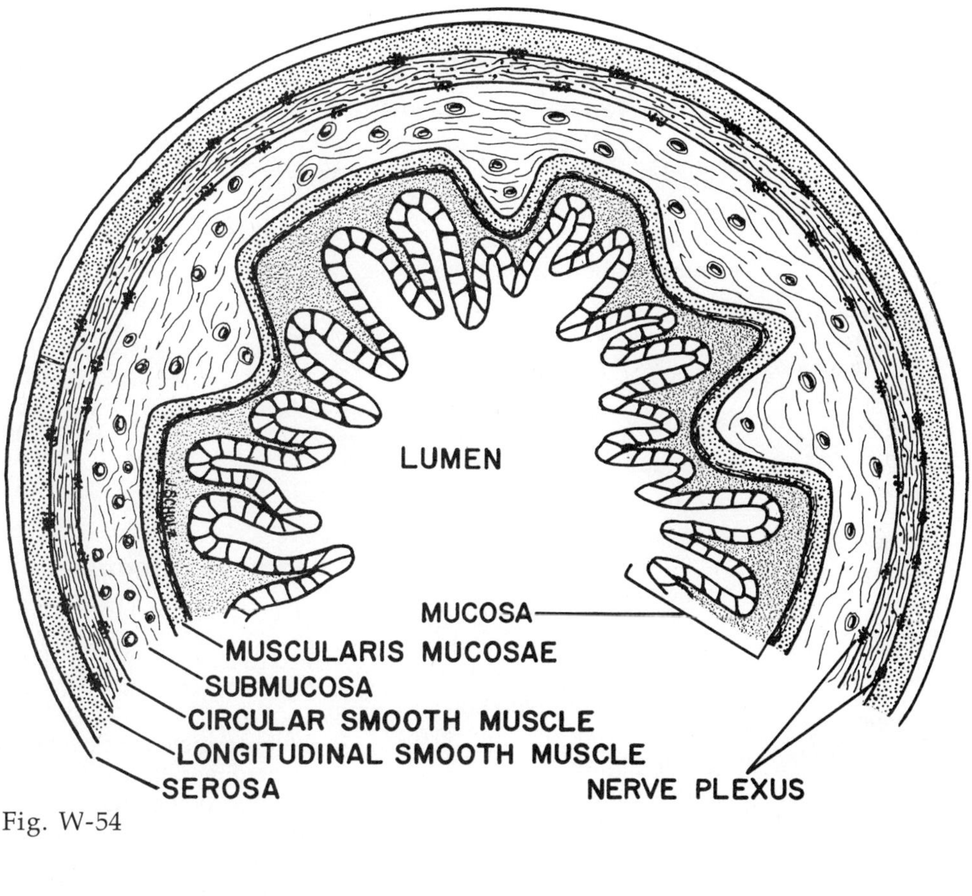

Fig. W-54

3. True. Other things may initiate salivation also, but stimulation of the receptors is the usual cause. *(361)*
4. False. Digestive activity *begins* in the mouth. *(360)*
5. True. The key word here is *control.* *(360)*
6. True. See answer 3 above. This is an example of the pressure receptors at work. *(361)*

7. True. Though we salivate most actively when eating, our salivary glands work continually to keep the mouth moist. This saliva is swallowed. (*361*)
8. False. Acid solutions such as lemon juice are the most potent stimuli. (*361*)
9. False. The gastroesophageal sphincter is the mechanism that is not fully developed in a newborn child and that causes regurgitation. (*362*)

Chapter 12: Module II

Part I

See Fig. 12-8, p. 363.

Part II

1. reduced lumps of food; a thick mixture of food particles and secreted fluids (*363*)
2. *a* external autonomic nerves
   b internal nerve plexuses
   c hormones secreted by the wall of the duodenum (*365*)
3. *a* continues to reduce large lumps of food to smaller ones
   b activates some of the enzymes secreted by the stomach
   c kills bacteria entering with food (*367*)
4. *a* distention of the duodenum
   b hypertonic solutions
   c acid
   d fat (*370*)
5. *a* walls of the duodenum (duodenal mucosa)
   b gastric mucosal layer (*371*)
6. *a* external autonomic nerves
   b internal nerve plexuses
   c hormones secreted by the GI tract (*371*)

Part III

1. *c* (*364–365*)
2. *a, c, d* (*365*)
3. *a, b, c, d* (*367*)
4. *b, c* (*367*)
5. *a* (*368*)
6. *b, c, d* (*370*)

Chapter 12: Module III

Part I

1. The cephalic phase of pancreatic secretions is controlled by the autonomic nerves to the pancreas, primarily the vagus nerve. (*375*)
2. *a* stimulates
   b inhibits
   c inhibits (*377*)
3. *Secretin:* causes an increase in bicarbonate secretion by the pancreas.
   CCK: causes an increase in enzyme secretion by the pancreas. (*376*)
4. *a* gallbladder
   b in liver cells (*376*)
5. Assuming it is functioning correctly, the pancreas is releasing more bicarbonate. (*376*)
6. *a* bile pigments
   b bile salts
   c cholesterol
   d lecithin (*376*)

Part II

1. True (*376*)
2. False. The presence of fat molecules in the duodenum stimulates the secretion of CCK. (*376*)
3. True (*378*)

Chapter 12: Module IV

Part I

1. segmentation (*379–380*)
2. *a* sodium
   b water
   c vitamins (or products synthesized by bacteria) (*388*)
3. See Fig. 12-27 and pp. 384–386, 387.

Part II

See Fig. 12-24, p. 383.

Part III

1. *a, b, c, d* (*380*)
2. *a, b, c* (*381*)
3. *a, d* (*381–384*)
4. *a, b, d* (*389–390*)

Chapter 13: Module 1

Part I

1. *d* (*397*)
2. protein (*397*)
3. *a, b, d* (*397–398*)
4. Glucose provides both the glycerol and fatty acid moieties of triglycerides which are synthesized in the liver by liver cells. (*394*)
5. *a, b* (*393–395*)

Part II

See Fig. 13-4, p. 394.

Chapter 13: Module II

Part I

1. True. The clusters of beta along with alpha (glucagon-producing) cells in the pancreas are known as the islets of Langerhans. *(398)*
2. False. Secretion of insulin is stimulated directly by elevated plasma glucose levels. *(400)*
3. True *(400)*
4. False. A lowered concentration of insulin is present during the postabsorptive state and causes increased permeability of cells only when in higher concentration. *(400)*
5. True. Ventilation will be increased by hydrogen ion stimulation of the medullary respiratory centers. High hydrogen ion concentration will be caused by dissociation of H^+ ions from the accumulation of fatty acids and ketone bodies. *(401)*
6. True *(401)*

Part II

1. *b, c, d* *(399)*
2. *a* *(401)*
3. *a, b, c* *(401)*

Chapter 13: Module III

Part I

1. True *(403)*
2. False. Epinephrine *stimulates* breakdown of TG in adipose tissue. *(403)*
3. True *(403)*
4. True *(402)*
5. False. Plasma glucose level is *low* during the postabsorptive period and higher during the absorptive period. *(403)*
6. True *(403)*
7. True *(403)*
8. True *(403)*
9. True *(403)*
10. False. It is controlled by the plasma glucose concentration. *(403)*
11. False. Plasma glucose concentration decreases in the presence of insulin. *(399)*

Part II

1. *a* (because insulin decreases the plasma glucose, which, in turn, stimulates GH secretion). *(406)*
2. *b, d* *(403–406)*
3. *a, c, d* *(403)*

Chapter 13: Module IV

Part I

1. False. Varies from organ to organ. *(406)*
2. True *(407)*
3. False. They affect many organs of the body. *(409)*
4. False. Not the nerves but some blood-borne agent appears responsible. *(410)*

Part II

1. *c* *(409)*
2. *a* *(407)*
3. *b* *(409)*
4. *d* *(406)*

Chapter 13: Module V

Part I

1. *a, b, c, d, e, f, g, h* *(412)*
2. *g, h* *(418–420)*

Part II

1. Food intake
   = heat production
   + external work
   = total energy expenditure

   (Since a steady state is involved, there is no net change in energy storage.) *(411, 414)*
2. Specific dynamic action
   = increase in metabolic rate due to ingestion of food. *(412)*
3. $\Delta E = \Delta$ heat $+ \Delta$ work *(410)*
4. See p. 411 and Fig. 13-22, p. 412.

Chapter 13: Module VI

Part I

1. *a, b* (Our basal metabolic rate does not increase but our metabolic rate does.) *(426)*
2. *b, c, d* *(426–427)*

Part II

1. False. Part of acclimatization to heat is lower sodium content in sweat to reduce excessive salt loss. *(426)*
2. True. This reduces blood flow to the surface and thus increases the insulating capacity of the skin. *(424)*
3. False. The fever is caused by elevation of the hypothalamic "set point." *(428–429)*
4. False. During an infection leading to a fever, our ability to regulate body temperature is not altered; we regulate our body temperature at a higher level. *(428)*

5. True. This in turn is thought to lower the hypothalamic "set point," reducing the fever. (*429*)

Chapter 14: Module I

Part I

See Fig. 14-5, p. 434, and Fig. 14-1, p. 432, for correct labels.

Part II

1. *a, c, d, e, f* (*437*)
2. *e, f* (*436*)
3. *a, b, c, d* (*436–437*)
4. *a* (*437*)
5. *a, b* (*438*)
6. *a, c* (*435*)
7. *a, b, d* (*431, 433, 436*)
8. *a, d* (*435*)
9. *b* (*435*)

Part III

1. orgasm (*435*)
2. primary spermatocyte secondary spermatocyte (*432*)
3. impotence (*435*)
4. between seminiferous tubules (*436*)
5. sperm, fluid from epithelium of epididymis, fluid from glands (seminal vesicles, prostate, and others) containing fructose and prostaglandins (*433–434*)

Chapter 14: Module II

Part I

1. *b* (*446*)
2. *b* (*443*)
3. *a, b, c* (*445*)
4. *c* (*446*)

Part II

1. False. Androgens. (*448*)
2. True (*446*)
3. False. Remains constant during the follicular phase with a large increase with corpus luteum development. (*443*)
4. True (*447*)
5. False. It is the fall in progesterone and estrogen that results in menstruation. (*446*)
6. False. Zona pellucida. (*439*)
7. True (*440*)

Part III

See Fig. 14-14, p. 443.

Part IV

See Fig. 14-11, p. 440. The site of secretion of estrogen is the follicle cells.

Chapter 14: Module III

Part I

See Fig. W-74, p. 269. Times of movement: (*a*) about 30 min; (*b*) within 10–15 hr; (*c*) about seven days. (*449–450*)

Part II

See Fig. W-75, p. 269. (*450, 453–455*)

Part III

1. *a, d*
2. *a, h*
3. *f, g*
4. *a, h*
5. *g*
6. *b* (*456–457*)

Part IV

1. True (*450*)
2. False (*450*)
3. False (induces ovulation) (*453*)

Chapter 14: Module IV

Part I

1. *c, d* (*443, 460*)
2. *b, d* (*460*)
3. *a, e* (*437, 445–446, 448, 458–460*)

Part II

1. An alteration in brain function leads to the release of increased amounts of releasing factors controlling FSH and LH secretion. Increase in these gonadotropins raises the secretion of testosterone and estrogen. (*464–465*)
2. It is the presence or absence of testosterone which determines early sexual development. (*464*)
3. With age there occurs a decrease in testicular function and a corresponding decrease in testosterone. With less negative feedback there is also an increase in gonadotropin levels. (*467*)

Part III

1. False. Refers to cutting of the oviducts. (suppl.)
2. True (*462–463*)
3. False. Gonadotropin release is unaffected. (*460*)
4. True (*466*)
5. False. Sterility refers to infertility, while impotence is the inability to achieve an erection. (*435*)

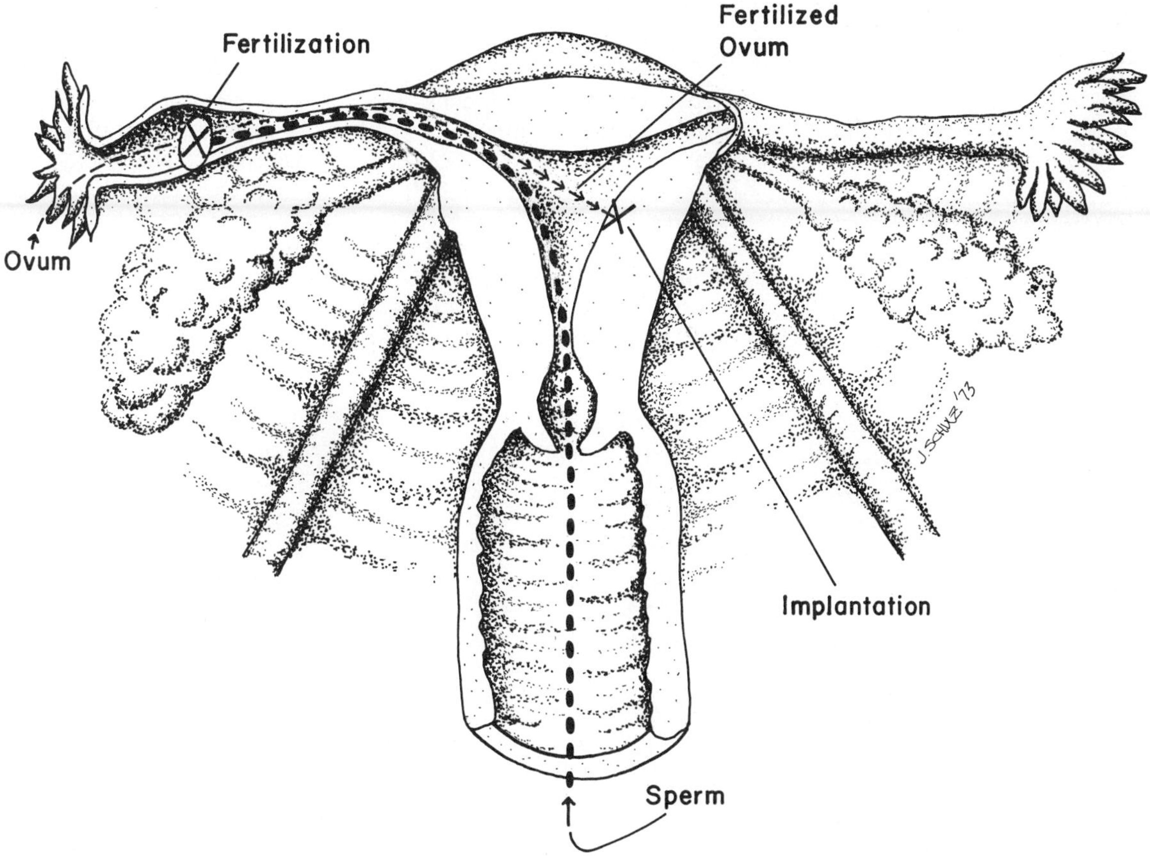

Fig. W-74

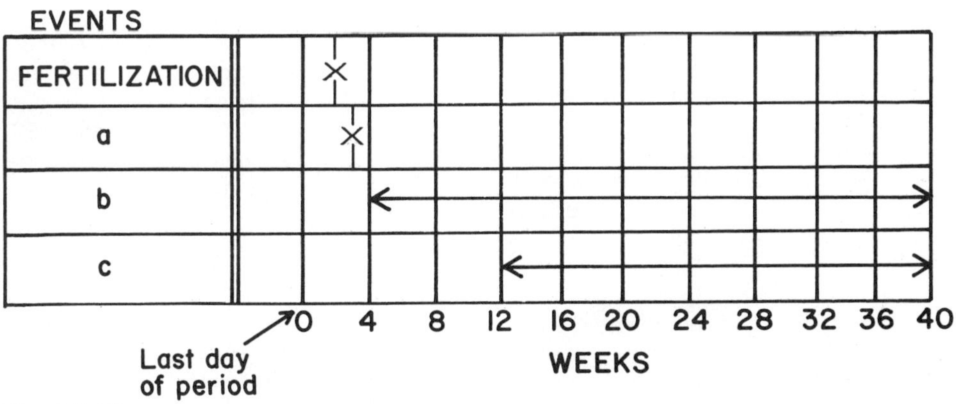

Fig. W-75

Chapter 15: Module I

Part I

1. *a* loss of vessel continuity
   b a greater pressure inside the vessel than outside (*468*)
2. thrombin (*471*)
3. megakaryocytes (*470*)
4. serotonin, epinephrine (*471*)

Part II

1. True (*469–470*)
2. True (*474*)
3. False. Plasmin and heparin. (*475*)

Part III

1. Venous bleeding is less dangerous because of the vein's low hydrostatic pressure. (*469*)
2. The tissues contain a substance known as tissue thromboplastin which can substitute for both platelet phospholipid and several of the plasma factors. This is known as the extrinsic clotting pathway. (*474*)
3. *a* platelets: colorless corpuscles that originate from large cells called megakaryocytes, that contain numerous granules and lack a nucleus. (*470*)
   b serum: plasma without fibrinogen. (*474*)
   c thrombosis: the presence of a thrombus or clot in a blood vessel. (*475*)
   d emboli: a plug (clot, air, etc.) present within a blood vessel. (*476*)

Chapter 15: Module II

Part I

1. nonspecific defense mechanisms, specific immune mechanisms (*477*)
2. lymphoid (*477*)
3. antibodies (*477*)
4. granulocytes, lymphocytes, monocytes, macrophages, plasma cells (*477*)
5. bone marrow (*477*)
6. *a* direct cellular destruction via enzymes
   b release toxins
   c drain host's energy supply
   d capture cell's metabolic and reproductive machinery (cancer?) (*477*)

Part II

1. True (*477*)
2. False. It is specific immunity that relies on the lymphoid cells. (*477*)
3. False. In the interstitial fluid. (*477*)

Part III

1. Humoral immunity is mediated by circulating antibodies; cell-mediated immunity is mediated by sensitized lymphocytes. (*477*)
2. *a* immunity: all the physiological mechanisms which allow the body to recognize foreign materials and to neutralize or eliminate them. (*476*)
   b monocytes: a type of leukocyte produced by the bone marrow, larger than granulocytes and with a single oval or horseshoe-shaped nucleus and relatively few cytoplasmic granules. Upon entering an infected area they are converted into macrophages. (*478*)
   c lymphocytes: a type of leukocyte, responsible for specific immunity with relatively large nucleus and scanty surrounding cytoplasm. The progeny of one type of lymphocyte differentiate into plasma cells. (*478*)

Chapter 15: Module III

Part I

1. *a* 5
   b 7
   c 1
   d 6
   e 4
   f 2
   g 3 (*480*)
2. brings plasma proteins and phagocytes into an area to enable destruction of microbes and tissue repair (*480*)
3. histamine, kinins (*481*)
4. neutrophil exudation, or the movement of neutrophils into the inflamed area (*482–483*)
5. mast cells, circulating basophils, platelets (*481*)

Part II

1. True (*481*)
2. False. Found in many different tissues of the body as well. (*481*)

3. False. These two tissues are incapable of cell division in adults. *(484)*

Part III

1. The neutrophils that are active in the inflammatory response release a protein which resets the hypothalamic thermostat at an elevated level. *(485)*
2. phagocytosis *(484)*
3. leukocytosis: It is a marked increase in the synthesis and release of neutrophils by the bone marrow. *(486)*
4. *a* chemotaxis is the attraction of living matter to an area by a certain chemical. (Can be neutrophils to an inflamed area) *(483)*
   b interferon is a nonspecific defense mechanism against viral infection. It is a protein which inhibits viral growth and replication and can be produced by different cell types of the body in response to a viral infection of the particular cell. *(486)*
   c an abscess is a bag of pus (containing microbes, leukocytes, and liquefied debris) walled off by fibroblasts and collagen *(484)*
   d a granuloma consists of numerous layers of phagocytic-type cells which have engulfed the microbial or nonmicrobial substance but cannot digest them. The granuloma is usually surrounded by a fibrous capsule. *(484)*

Chapter 15: Module IV

Part I

1. True *(486)*
2. True *(487)*
3. True *(495)*
4. False. For many microorganisms the memory component of the antibody does not occur. *(493)*
5. False. They confer specific immune resistance against most bacteria. *(488)*
6. True *(493)*

Part II

1. gamma globulins immunoglobulins *(489)*
2. complement *(491)*
3. antigen-antibody complexes *(490)*

Part III

1. plasma, antibody *(492–493)*
2. By combining chemically with them, thus preventing the interaction of the toxin with susceptible cell membrane sites. *(492)*
3. Interfering with the synthesis of the bacteria's production of some essential macro molecule. *(495)*
4. Active immunity is the resistance which is built up as a result of actual contact with microorganisms and their toxins or other antigenic components, but passive immunity is the direct transfer of actively formed antibodies from one person or animal to another. *(493–494)*
5. Antibody is a specialized protein capable of combining chemically with the specific antigen which stimulated its production. *(488)*

Chapter 15: Module V

Part I

1. *a, c* *(498)*
2. *a, c* *(496)*
3. *d* *(497)*

Part II

1. True *(497)*
2. False. No one develops them unless exposed to Rh-type cells from another person. *(497)*
3. False. T cells. *(496)*
4. True *(499)*
5. True *(496)*

Part III

1. A, B, and O *(497)*
2. *a* The recipient's anti-B antibody causes the transfused cells to be attacked.
   b The anti-A antibody in the transfused plasma causes the recipient's cells to be attacked. *(497)*
3. *a* alteration of normal antigens
   b infection with a virus leading to production of new antigens
   c genetic mutations leading to new antigens
   d similarities of microbe's antigens with our own antigenic molecules
   e exposure of certain tissues (and their antigens) which had not previously been exposed to organs responsible for recognizing self-antigens *(499)*

Chapter 15: Module VI

Part I

1. Secretion of cortisol and activity of the sympathetic

nervous system are usually increased. (499)
2. pharmacological effects (501)
3. Hypothalamus secretes ACTH-releasing factor into the portal vessels in response to stress signals reaching various regions of brain. ACTH-RF stimulates ACTH release from anterior pituitary. ACTH in turn stimulates the adrenal cortex to release cortisol. (500)

Part II

1. *a* (501)
2. *b, c, d* (501)
3. *a* (500–501)

Part III

1. False. By many body cells, not by the brain. (500)
2. True (502)
3. True (500)

Part IV

1, 3, 4, 5, 6, 8 (502)

Chapter 16: Module I

Part I

1. *a, b, c* (507)
2. *a* L, I
   b I
   c I, L
   d L, I
   e L
   f L (506–507)
3. *e* (504)

Part II

1. sensory unit (504)
2. receptive field (504)
3. lateral inhibition (507)
4. nonspecific (504)
5. quantity (506)

Part III

1. False. This describes stimulus quality, not quantity. (504–505)
2. False. Sensory information is only that segment of the total afferent input which has a conscious correlate, i.e., a conscious awareness of the physical world. (503)
3. False. Sight, hearing, and possibly taste are not represented in the somatosensory cortex. (508)
4. True (506)
5. False. There is a gradient and therefore the pattern information is great. In fact, this is an important mechanism of stimulus location. (507)
6. True (507)

Chapter 16: Module II

Part I

1. True (509)
2. False. Signals changes in pressure. (509)
3. False. There is a mixture, i.e., some fire this way, and some do just the opposite. (509)
4. True (509)
5. False. Do not know how cold receptors function. (509)
6. False. This can be done by drugs or operation on the brain, interrupting pathways connecting the frontal lobe of the cerebrum with other brain parts. (510)
7. False. Only a small portion, between 400–700 nanometers (visible light). (511)
8. False. Lens changes shape. (512)
9. True (512)
10. False. Shift is from cone to rod receptors. (515)
11. True (516)
12. True (518)

Part II

1. *d* (509)
2. *b, c, d, e, f* (509)
3. *a, b* (510)
4. *a, d, e, f* (510)
5. *e* (511)
6. *b* (518)

Part III

1. accommodation (512)
2. I *c*
   II *d*
   III *b, c*
   IV *a, d*
   V *e*
   VI *a, b, c, d, e*
   VII *b, c*
   VIII *a, d* (512)
3. I R, C
   II R
   III R
   IV C
   V R
   VI C
   VII R, C (514–515)
4. I 6
   II 4
   III 1
   IV 2
   V 7
   VI 5
   VII 3 (515)
5. simple (518)
6. complex (518)

7. complex (*518*)
8. *a* search for visual targets
   b tracking of visual objects
   c compensation for movements of the head
   d convergence (*521*)
9. I *e*
   II *a*
   III *b*
   IV *d* (*521*)

Chapter 16: Module III

Part I

1. I *c*
   II *a, d*
   III *b* (*523*)
2. I *d*
   II *d*
   III *c*
   IV *a*
   V *f* (523–524)
3. I *5*
   II *6*
   III *1*
   IV 3
   V 4
   VI 2
   VII 7 (*523–524*)
4. comparison of times of stimulus onset and perception of relative intensity of sound at each ear (*526*)
5. motion; position of head (*526*)
6. *a* semicircular canals
   b utricule and saccule (*528*)

Part II

1. *b, c, e, f, g, h* (*524*)
2. *b, c, d, f* (*524*)
3. *a, b, c, d* (*526*)
4. *b, c, d, f, g* (*526*)
5. *b, c, d* (*530*)
6. *a, c, d, f, g, h* (*532*)

Part III

1. False. Total force is the same, but since the area of the oval window is 15 to 20 times smaller than the area of the tympanic membrane, the pressure (per unit area) is 15 to 20 times greater. (*524*)
2. False. Most impulses pass to the scala vestibuli and are transmitted to the basilar membrane which then deflects into the scala tympanic. (*524*)
3. True (*524*)
4. False. Found in the utricle and in the saccule, not in the semicircular canals. (*528*)
5. True (*528*)
6. True (*528*)
7. False. A single receptor cell can respond in varying degrees to many different substances falling into more than one of the basic categories. In fact, this is important in determining the quality of the taste sensation. (*531*)
8. True (*531*)
9. True (*531*)
10. True (*532*)
11. False. There are no differences in cells, but meaningful differences between receptors are thought to exist on a molecular level, i.e., odor discrimination depends upon different types of interactions between the odor-substance molecules and receptor sites. Simultaneous yet differential stimulation of many receptor cells provides the basis for discrimination. (*532*)

Chapter 16: Module IV

Part I

1. primary (visual) cortex or somatosensory cortex (*532*)
2. cortical association cortex (*532*)
3. I A
   II S
   III A
   IV A
   V A (*532–533*)
4. I *b*
   II *a*
   III *a*
   IV *b*
   V *a*
   VI *b* (*533–534*)

Part II

1. False. Sensory input is a function of signals from receptors and cannot be learned. (*534*)
2. True (*534*)
3. True (*533*)
4. True (*533*)

Part III

1. *a, c, d, e, f* (*533–534*)

Chapter 17: Module I

Part I

1. *b, d* (*537–538*)
2. *a, b, c* (*541*)
3. *a, b* (*538*)

Part II

1. reciprocal innervation (*540–541*)
2. alpha motor neurons (*541*)
3. gamma motor neurons (*541*)

Part III

1. False. They are not the same; gamma innervates spindles and alpha innervates skeletomotor. (*541*)
2. True (*541*)
3. False. Higher brain centers. (*538*)
4. True (*540*)
5. False. Monosynaptic. (*540*)

Chapter 17: Module II

Part I

1. *a, c, d* (*545*)
2. *a, b, c* (*545–546*)
3. *a, b, d* (*548*)
4. *b, c, d* (*549*)

Part II

1. *a* receptor
   b afferent pathway
   c integrating center (CNS)
   d efferent pathway
   e effector (*126*)
2. pyramidal tract or pyramidal system (*545*)
3. intention tremor or oscillating tremor (*547*)

Part III

1. False. In the right half of the brain. (*545*)
2. True (*545*)
3. True (*547*)

Chapter 18: Module I

Part I

See Fig. 18-1, p. 554, for correct answers.

Part II

1. *a* (*555*)
2. *a, b, d* (*556–557*)

Chapter 18: Module II

Part I

1. short-term memory (*566*)
2. aphasia (*568*)
3. long-term memory (*566*)

Part II

1. *a, b, c* (*561*)
2. *a* (*561–563*)
3. *d* (*569*)
4. *b* (*560*)
5. *b* (*569*)
6. *a, b, c* (*565*)